MY VENUS FLYTRAP
WON'T OPEN

Laura - thank you for your support, enjoy!

Danielle D...

MY VENUS FLYTRAP WON'T OPEN

DANIELLE DUMAIS

NEW DEGREE PRESS

MY VENUS FLYTRAP WON'T OPEN

ISBN   978-1-63676-530-3   *Paperback*

978-1-63676-071-1   *Kindle Ebook*

978-1-63676-072-8   *Ebook*

"*If sexuality is one dimension of our ability to live passionately…then in cutting off our sexual feelings we diminish our overall power to feel, know, and value deeply.*"

—JUDITH PLASKOW

Contents

Introduction

They're giggling and lying on the carpeted floor. One drink too many and, well, that's where they ended up. By their feet, a pink splotch from spilled punch someone tried and failed to scrub away remains disastrously obvious against the white carpet. That, and other sloppy sloshing throughout the evening, have left the room smelling faintly of a distillery mixed with the heady scents of two dozen different flowery perfumes.

It's the Fourth of July, but the fireworks haven't started yet so everyone at the party is mingling inside the stuffy apartment, their voices growing louder as cheap alcohol fills them. But the cloud of noise barely registers with the two women lying shoulder to shoulder amidst throngs of legs.

Lost in their own bubble, their giggles turn to harsher scoffs as the conversation strikes a more serious chord. It hardly seems the time to bring it up, but booze has a way of loosening tongues and trust has a way of coaxing out hidden truths.

Inhaling and turning her blue eyes on her friend, Savannah says, "It doesn't work for me either. Sex, I mean. It hurts too much, just like with you." As her friend takes in her confession and begins profusely pontificating over their shared vagina woes, Savannah feels a glimmer of relief bloom in her chest.

From the outset, you wouldn't know there was anything at all amiss with twenty-two-year-old Savannah. Raised in a bustling North Carolina town, traces of southern charm evident in her bubbly personality, she always has a smile reserved for anyone.

But Savannah suffers from an invisible illness. Invisible, not only because she lacks a physical sign or mark on her body, but also because Savannah has largely kept her ailment hidden even from those closest to her.

Suffering physically and mentally, why would she choose to keep this a secret?

She knew something was off, but she didn't know what and was too embarrassed to look for further help. Savannah began to feel as if something was wrong with her, thought she wasn't "normal." No one else she knew seemed to have these issues, and she didn't know who she could turn to about such a sensitive topic.

Savannah didn't know the pain she was experiencing was actually a sexual dysfunction disorder—not only very real, but something many other women suffer with in silence. This, and many other female sexual health issues, are not discussed or taught in sex ed classes, are not widely known in the general public, and are even a mystery to some physicians.

Back on the floor of the party, Savannah felt the tension roll from her shoulders as she spilled her secret. But as the warm fuzziness from the alcohol faded from her brain, and the lingering guests stole away back to their respective homes, her reality confronted her again. Alone and sober, she tucked it back deep inside her body, like a splinter in her finger which needled her every time she started to forget it was there. Better to just ignore it. It was easier and much less scary this way. Better to just pretend she was "normal."

In the world of sexual education and sexual health, it may seem as if we've come a long way since the first studies of human sexual behaviors began in earnest with researcher Alfred Kinsey in the late 1940s and early 1950s.[1] Well into the twenty-first century, we have a robust sex-positive movement in the US which claims to educate and empower everyone to explore their sexuality and promote consensual sexual expression. The movement, which gained traction as part of the second-wave feminist movement in the 80s, paved the way for conversations about consent, self-defined sexuality, gender myths, safe sex, rape culture, and body positivity. It has been a way for people who have historically been sexually oppressed, victimized, or hyper-sexualized, to embrace their sexuality and sexual well-being.

Historically, our culture has reserved sexual empowerment, encouragement, and satisfaction for cisgender, heterosexual,

---

1 Brown Theodore, and Elizabeth Fee, "Alfred C. Kinsey: A Pioneer Of Sex Research," *American journal of public health* 93, no. 6 (June 2003): 896-897; *Science and Its Times: Understanding the Social Significance of Scientific Discovery*, s.v. "The Study of Human Sexuality," accessed August 21, 2020.

white men. The sex-positivity movement, however, has grown over the past few decades to encompass a broader scope of human sexuality, gender identities, races, and classes. Within the umbrella of sex positivity, women's health has additionally seen great progress since Margaret Sanger first started the fight for women's rights to birth control in the early 1900s.[2]

Second-wave feminism activists brought forth the Women's Health Movement in the 1960s and 70s with the goal of assuming autonomy over their sexual health and liberating themselves from a "paternalistic and condescending medical community."[3] But while the sex-positive movement is grounded in inclusivity and sex positivity for all, it fails to extend to the sexual health sphere.

How is it leaving some behind?

It begins with sex ed. The rhetoric regarding sexual health or sex when we are growing up, especially for teenage girls, is often risk-, fear-, and pain-based. Our sexual education in middle and high schools, if we are afforded it, is premised on the ways in which we can keep ourselves healthy by mitigating the negative sides or outcomes of sex.

---

2   D. Wardell, "Margaret Sanger: birth control's successful revolutionary," *American journal of public health* 70, no. 7 (July 1980): 736-742.

3   Francine Nichols, "History of the Women's Health Movement in the 20th Century," *Journal of Obstetric, Gynecologic & Neonatal Nursing* 29, no. 1 (June 1999): 56-64; M.S. Geary, "An analysis of the women›s health movement and its impact on the delivery of health care within the United States," *Nurse Practitioner* 20, no. 11 PT 1 (1995): 24-27.

Conversely, when we enter adulthood, we are faced with a sex positivity sphere which likes to focus on the sexually healthy, the sexually normal, and the sexually pleasing, with a very narrow definition and view of what constitutes a healthy, normal, positive sex life.

As a result, women are programmed to expect the worst from sex as we go through adolescence until we reach a point when those expectations flip. Suddenly, sex is what everyone's talking about and according to the sex-positive movement, sex should be just as amazing for women.

Yes, "ladies," let's claim our sexual pleasure.

But because there isn't often a balance of understanding between the risks and the benefits of sex, nor are we often encouraged to talk about our own sexual well-being, a lot of women miss their sexual health warning signs.

In fact, sex education for tweens and teens is so focused on prevention—preventing girls from acting too promiscuous, from being sexually active, from getting pregnant—rather than honest and open discussion, we are woefully unprepared to deal with our own sexual health. We haven't been taught our healthy sexuality is an important part of who we are.

I received quite an extensive sexual education growing up: my mom took me out of middle school health class because she thought the curriculum was not comprehensive enough and taught me herself. I also attended, much to my chagrin, a fourteen-week sex ed course at my church for three hours every Sunday night which covered everything from consent to how to put a condom on a cucumber.

Yet, though my sex ed addressed healthy sex practices, and wasn't so naive to assume abstinence is the be-all-end-all, I still found myself missing crucial information.

Those gaps in education followed me into young adulthood, into college life rife with so-called "hookup culture." I, like so many other teenage girls experiencing "abnormal" sexual health challenges, missed my early warning signs. Too uncomfortable to talk to my physician and met with confusion from friends and family when I mentioned anything, I decided to pretend nothing was wrong. Quite literally pushing through my issues, it gradually began to take a toll on my mental health, as well as my physical health.

The day I finally got answers from my doctor was a day of mixed emotions. It was news I didn't want to hear, but at the same time, it was news I wished I had received many years prior. My experiences showed me there is a lot we don't talk about when it comes to female sexual health, and the ways in which many sex ed classes are framed leave certain individuals vulnerable to untreated health issues, discrimination, and unhealthy views of sexuality and bodily autonomy.

The stories in this book from the incredibly brave women and assigned female at birth (AFAB) individuals who shared their experiences with me aim to illustrate the consequences of allowing sexual health issues and sexuality conversations to slip through the cracks.

Their stories reinforce the narrative that generalizing sexual health and sexuality perpetuates stereotypes and misinformation:

- Safe sex is not always synonymous with positive sex
- The tendency to contextualize women's bodies in relation to someone else, rather than recognizing their individual sexual health needs irrespective of a partner, can ultimately have damaging effects
- Many aspects of sexual health are still overlooked in the "sex-positive" movement, including:
  - sexual dysfunction
  - sexual trauma
  - and low sexual desire.

To have full inclusivity in the sex-positive campaign, we must break down the remaining barriers which leave women feeling broken, silenced, and invisible. Barriers that include ignoring very valid concerns simply because they make others feel uncomfortable.

I want to understand how to bring the principles of sex positivity to those who have been excluded by bringing these issues to the forefront. Sex positivity is a human rights issue overlooking many, many people. Shedding a light on those people and their experiences is crucial to improve the sexual well-being of emerging generations.

The goal of this book is to reach women dealing with these "invisible" illnesses. I want to show them they are not alone. They are not forgotten. They deserve to have their voices heard at the sex-positive table.

As these stories reach not only these women but educators, health care professionals, and parents as well, they will help fill a gap in sex education, prompting dialogue and promoting greater acceptance and a more comprehensive understanding of female sexuality and sexual health.

PART 1

UNCOVERING THE ROOTS

CHAPTER 1

Sex Positivity: A Brief History

What is sex positivity?

When I first started hearing about sex positivity, I associated it with casual sex and hookup culture: a magazine article spouting the "6 Yoga Poses for Better Sex" and Instagram influencers reviewing the best new vibrators to hit the market. I thought of lingerie ads and women unboxing their stories of fake orgasms. I thought of sex positivity as moving the sex conversation from its dingy, dusty little corner to center stage. Glitzy, glamorous, and glorified, a great sex life is like a fashion accessory—an aesthetic, an achievement.

But sex positivity isn't just about saying, "Yes!" to sex. There are many definitions of the sex-positive ideology, but at its core, the movement was born in response to sex negativity, or viewing sex as something shameful, dirty, and damaging. It wanted to do the opposite: approach sex as a healthy, vibrant, joyful part of life.

The sex-positive trend began challenging "sexual morals" and repressive norms long before the so-called sexual revolution of the 1960s. Rapid urbanization in the early 1900s leading to the rise of "mass culture," public health nurse Margaret Sanger's birth control legalization campaign, and the advent of the notorious flapper girls swept the US into the roaring 20s and an uncharted sex culture.[4] A decade awash in jazz music, unchaperoned dancing, and sexual experimentation had social conservatives fearing for the loss of their pure American values.

Of particular concern to the social hygienists were the increasingly popular "petting parties," which encouraged casual physical indulgence between partners.[5] Akin to modern-day "hookup culture," petting parties became a staple of the 1920s and 1930s college and sometimes high school experience; similar to the term hookup, petting meant something different to everyone.[6] For teenagers and young adults, these parties provided a safe way for them to explore their sexuality with clear limits. The exploration would stop before intercourse to preserve virginity and prevent sexually transmitted infections (STIs).[7]

Around the same time, a wave of slightly wilder parties home to drag queens, raunchy songs, and celebrities blossomed in New York City.[8] Known as the "Pansy Craze," these

4   "The Roaring Twenties History," History, last modified August 12, 2020; "A Brief History of Birth Control in the U.S.," Our Bodies Our Selves, last modified July 8, 2020.

5   Linton Weeks, "When 'Petting Parties' Scandalized The Nation," NPR, May 16, 2015; Erin Blakemore, "The Scandalous Sex Parties That Made Americans Hate Flappers," History, last modified July 21, 2019.

6   Blakemore, "Scandalous Sex Parties.

7   Weeks, "When 'Petting Parties.'"; Blakemore, "Scandalous Sex Parties."

8   Darryl W. Bullock, "Pansy Craze: the wild 1930s drag parties that kickstarted gay nightlife," The Guardian, September 14, 2017; Lisa Hix, "Singing the Lesbian Blues in 1920s Harlem," Collectors Weekly, July 9, 2013.

balls have roots stretching back to 1869 Harlem, but rose to elevated popularity in the 1920s during the Harlem Renaissance.[9] The "Pansy and Lesbian Craze" grew out of the advent of LGBTQ+ communities and spaces in Harlem pioneered largely by black queer women.

As blues and jazz took over the music scene of New York, queer individuals found their voices in the "sexually freewheeling" lyrics of the genre which allowed for a rare freedom of expression for same-sex desires in the relative sanctuary of theater and night club culture.[10] Black blues women like Bessie Smith and Ma Rainey used the entertainment platform to publicly portray themselves as "explicitly sexual beings" through their stage personae, eventually exposing mainstream society to messages of alternative sexuality and growing an active—albeit clandestine—LGBTQ+ enclave.[11] Black, queer, blues women challenging traditional ideas about love and openly flouting their sexuality progressed the gay liberation movement and helped shape mainstream culture far beyond the streets of Harlem.[12]

---

9   Bullock, "Pansy Craze."
10   Emma Chen, "Black Face, Queer Space: The Influence of Black Lesbian & Transgender Blues Women of the Harlem Renaissance on Emerging Queer Communities," *Historical Perspectives: Santa Clara University Undergraduate Journal of History, Series II* 21, no. 8 (2016): 20-21; Terry Rowden, "Harlem Undercover: Difference and Desire in African American Popular Music, 1920-1940," *English Language Notes* 45, no. 2 (October 2007): 23.
11   Chen, "Black Face," 21, 22, 27; "T'ain't nobody's bizness: queer blues divas of the 1920's," directed by Robert Philipson (2011; San Francisco, CA: Shoga Films) DVD.
12   Chen, "Black Face," 22, 26, 25; Angela Y. Davis, *Blues Legacies and Black Feminism: Gertrude Ma Rainey, Bessie Smith, and Billie Holiday* (New York: Vintage Books, 1999), 103; Hix, "Singing.

Petting parties, blues music and the move toward a sexually "freer" culture arose both in response to a stifling Victorian-era society which imposed strict sexual regulations and as a natural response to the end of a repressive World War I environment.[13] But the Jazz Age also saw the surge of organized counter movements aimed at suppressing sexual experimentation, cleansing away the evils of sexual promiscuity, and preserving the conservative American way of life. Organizations such as the League of American Women and the Women's Christian Temperance Union took it upon themselves to censor the behavior of America's youth, pinpointing the "immoral" flapper girls as wanton temptresses driving their boys, and American society, into the gutter.[14]

Although the Great Depression, a second world war, and the post-war suburbia boom promoting white-picket-fence family values dampened the flapper lifestyle and helped serve the societal safe guardians' goals, the sexual evolution wasn't finished. The sex-positive movement was not only driven by sexually curious, cigarette-smoking, slang-using college students. Sex positivity relies just as much on knowledge and information about the confusing world of sex as it does on acceptance, and up until the 1930s, the field of sex research was sorely lacking.

That began to change when, in 1938, biology professor and researcher Alfred Kinsey agreed to teach a course on marriage and family at Indiana University.[15] As a part of his

---

13   Weeks, "When 'Petting Parties.'"
14   Ibid.
15   Theodore M. Brown and Elizabeth Fee, "Alfred C. Kinsey: A Pioneer Of Sex Research," *American Journal of Public Health* 93, no. 6 (June 2003): 896.

course, Kinsey taught extensively on the biology of sexual stimulation, the mechanical workings of intercourse, how to use contraception, and criticized social attitudes about what constituted normal sexual behavior.[16]

As one of his biographers James H. Jones writes, Kinsey leveraged his marriage course to "transform his private struggle against Victorian morality into a public crusade," to which his students responded eagerly.[17] But Kinsey's truly revolutionary work came from his research studies on human sexual behavior, the first comprehensive and objective sex behavior studies conducted utilizing the scientific method.

Before Kinsey's work, sex research was largely subject to personal bias and misleading information. During the nineteenth and well into the twentieth century, physicians were considered the experts on the topic of sexology despite having no specialized knowledge in the field. Homosexuality and masturbation were classified as deviant behavior or a sign of mental illness by psychiatrists and the public alike.[18] Kinsey's two books (*Sexual Behavior in the Human Male* and *Sexual Behavior in the Human Female*), which helped to dispel myths about masturbation, homosexuality, premarital

---

16 Ibid.
17 James H. Jones, *Alfred C. Kinsey: A Public/Private Life* (New York: W. W. Norton & Company, 1997), quoted in Theodore M. Brown and Elizabeth Fee, "Alfred C. Kinsey: A Pioneer Of Sex Research," *American Journal of Public Health* 93, no. 6 (June 2003): 896.
18 *Science and Its Times: Understanding the Social Significance of Scientific Discovery*, s.v. "The Study of Human Sexuality," accessed August 21, 2020

intercourse, and how sex plays a part in the lives of women, also petitioned other researchers to take up the torch.[19]

For example, Evelyn Hooker, one of the most prominent champions of normalizing homosexuality, conducted a 1957 study called "The Adjustment of the Male Overt Homosexual" which caused the American Psychiatric Academy to reevaluate the classification of homosexuality as a mental illness.[20] Paralleling the start of the sexual revolution in the 60s came William Masters' and Virginia Johnson's studies on the physiological aspects of human sexuality, which explored sexual arousal and orgasm and spearheaded the field of sex therapy.[21]

The advances in sex research and a broadening public understanding of sexuality paved the way for the sexual revolution of the 60s and early 70s, but what truly differentiated these decades from other sexual radicalism periods in the US was the creation and rollout of the birth control pill in 1960 and the legalization of abortion in 1973.[22]

What with second-wave feminism and an era saturated with youth counterculture issues like racial integration and anti-war protests, conservative America was in societal upheaval. Nothing rocked the "moralists'" boats more than the lurking threat of gender equality and female

---

19 Ibid.
20 Ibid.
21 Ibid.
22 "A Brief History of Birth Control," Our Bodies Our Selves; Nancy L. Cohen, *Delirium: The Politics of Sex in America* (Berkley, CA: Counterpoint, 2012), 9.

sexual liberation, forces guaranteed to tarnish their carefully sanitized social fabric. Conservative organizations like the Moral Majority, the Eagle Forum, and Operation Rescue sprang up to defend the country from what they felt was a vicious attack on traditional American family values and morals.[23]

The ideas concerning sex and sexuality were changing: "Sex was no longer a source of consternation but a cause for celebration; its presence not what made a person morally suspect, but rather its absence."[24] But sex, according to the moralists, was sinful and corrupting—something to be done just between a husband and wife to create a child, not something to be trivialized as an act of pleasure.

Sixty years later, in the decade of 2020, the messages of "sex is demoralizing" are evident in raging abortion battles, abstinence-only sex ed, and the debasement of sexual assault victims underscored by the exoneration of their perpetrators. In 2019 alone, Republican-led states passed fifty-nine abortion restrictions, and according to a 2017 Department of Justice survey, out of every one thousand sexual assaults, fewer than five perpetrators will be incarcerated.[25]

---

23 *Encyclopedia Britannica Online*, s.v. "Moral Majority," accessed August 31, 2020; "Eagle Forum Brochure," Eagle Forum, accessed August 31, 2020; "Who We Are," Operation Rescue, accessed August 31, 2020.

24 Rachel Hills, "What Every Generation Gets Wrong About Sex," *Time*, December 2, 2014.

25 Yelena Dzhanova, "The battle over abortion rights: Here's what's at stake in 2020," CNBC, last modified January 6, 2020; "National Crime Victimization Survey 2010-2016," Department of Justice Bureau of Justice Statistics, 2017, cited in "The Criminal Justice System: Statistics," Rape, Abuse & Incest National Network, accessed August 31, 2020.

But contemporary popular culture spins a different story. The messages in our music, TV, art, literature, and more are imbued with themes of casual, pleasurable sex. Leading a robust sex life is depicted as empowering, the key to a rich life, even a necessity for mental well-being. But sex-positive messages have grown more complex over the decades; it's not as easy as saying sex isn't dirty anymore. It's also not predicated on the fallacy more sex equals sex positivity. In fact, sexual guilt tied not to having sex, but rather to not having *enough* sex, is a contradiction from which the modern sexual freedom sphere is trying to move away.

The current sex positivity framework is based on the principles of personal freedom and choice—in other words, someone having full autonomy over their sexuality.[26] *The ideology rejects:*

- *rape culture*
- *slut-shaming*
- *kink-shaming*
- *gender stereotypes*
- and *homophobia.*

Instead, it encourages healthy sexual expression, whether that be:

- *people exploring their sexual identity*
- *participating in casual sex*
- *choosing to engage in polygamy*

---

26 Shruti Jani, "Since It's Rubbished So Much, What Exactly Is Sex-Positive Feminism?" Feminism in India, March 27, 2018.

- *or anything else that embraces the idea of mutually consensual and safe sex practices.*

One of the more radical and controversial aspects of the movement has been the challenging of gender stereotypes which equate biological sex to gender, place people in boxes, and ultimately bar someone from healthy sexual expression. The ideology rejects two gender-constraining concepts: male vilification and gender essentialism.

> *Male vilification, based on traditionally heteronormative standards, describes male sexuality as "aggressive, insatiable and a testosterone-fueled rampage."*[27]

Think "boys will be boys." This view aligns women's sexuality with suggestions of purity, chastity, and passivity. Male vilification strips women of their sexual interest and autonomy and promotes rape culture by justifying the behavior of sexually driven males.

These constrictive and limited ideas of the gender binary characterize men as the sexual beasts and conquerors who just can't help themselves, and paint women as having no vested interest in their own sexual experience. Women are responsible for fighting off the advances of the horny males to maintain our virtue, lest we succumb to corrupting forces which land us squarely in Whoreville.

---

27 Ibid.

The virgin/whore dichotomy and the hypocrisy behind rape culture rhetoric stem from the widely discredited concept of gender essentialism.

> *Gender essentialism: the belief that males and females are born with certain innate tendencies and traits which are determined biologically, rather than culturally.*[28]

Gender essentialism equates gender and sex and adheres to traditional gender roles which follow a strict gender binary.

> *Gender binary: a concept or belief there are only two genders and one's sex or gender assigned at birth will align with traditional social constructs of masculine and feminine identity, expression, and sexuality.*[29]

Many societies, traditionally, have viewed biological sex as a rigid binary (i.e. male or female) and translated that view to a binary understanding of gender.[30] But even at the anatomical and chromosomal levels, this is not true.

Intersex/difference of sexual development (DSD) traits exist, wherein a person is born with, or develops over time, sexual and reproductive anatomy which does not seem to fit into "typical" male or female classifications.[31] The existence of intersex/DSD individuals demonstrates

---

28 *Oxford Reference*, s.v. "gender essentialism," accessed June 2, 2020.
29 *Dictionary.com*, s.v. "gender binary," accessed September 7, 2020.
30 "Understanding Gender," Gender Spectrum, accessed September 7, 2020.
31 "What is intersex?" Intersex Society of North America accessed September 7, 2020.

a biological sex spectrum disproving the idea there are only two sexes.[32]

According to the Intersex Society of North America, "Intersex is a socially constructed category that reflects real biological variation...in human cultures, sex categories get simplified into male, female, and sometimes intersex, in order to simplify social interactions, express what we know and feel, and maintain order."[33]

It's not nature or biology determining whether someone is male or female, it's humans. We have created the idea of gender based off sex anatomy and chromosomes; just as genitalia is not binary, neither is gender identity. Sometimes one's gender identity does not align with their biological sex:

- A person whose personal and gender identity corresponds with their sex assigned at birth is **cisgender.**[34]
- A person whose personal and gender identity does not correspond with their sex assigned at birth is **transgender.**[35]
- A person whose personal and gender identity does not fall into the category of either "male" or "female" is most commonly known as **non-binary.**[36]

---

32 "Understanding Gender," Gender Spectrum.
33 "What is intersex?" Intersex Society of North America.
34 *Merriam-Webster*, s.v. "cisgender," accessed September 7, 2020.
35 *Merriam-Webster*, s.v. "transgender," accessed September 7, 2020.
36 "Understanding Non-Binary People: How to Be Respectful and Supportive," National Center for Transgender Equality, October 5, 2018.

Throughout this book, I use the terms women and assigned female at birth (AFAB). The term "woman" includes anyone who identifies as such, whether or not they have typical female anatomy. However, for some of the sexual health issues I discuss, the term "woman" is referring to cisgender women, as the health issues are unique to the uterine reproductive system. AFAB refers to individuals who were born with typical female anatomy, but who may not identify as women.

Promoting the ideas of gender essentialism and the gender binary negates the existence of non-binary and trans individuals. Sex-positive thought challenges restrictive gender norms which can typecast people in inappropriate and damaging ways.

Dismantling gender stereotypes allows for freer sexuality exploration, fluidity, and liberation. It encourages those outside of the white, cisgender, heterosexual, male standard to empower themselves sexually. Moreover, the sex positivity movement highlights the physical and emotional wellness which comes from a healthy view of one's sexuality, positioning sexual health as integral to an individual's overall well-being.

Sexual health: "a state of physical, emotional, mental and social well-being in relation to sexuality; it is not merely the absence of disease, dysfunction or infirmity. Sexual health requires a positive and respectful approach to sexuality and sexual relationships, as well as the possibility of having pleasurable and safe sexual experiences, free of coercion, discrimination and violence."[37]

---

37 World Health Organization, *Defining sexual health: Report of a technical consultation on sexual health 28–31 January 2002, Geneva* (Geneva: WHO, 2006), 5, accessed June 4, 2020.

The World Health Organization (WHO) also maintains an individual's sexual intimacy and orientation enhance the individual's personality, communication, and love.[38]

Presenting sexual health as a critical factor in an individual's general physical and emotional health presents crucial questions:

- What about those who are chronically sexually dysfunctional?
- What about those who are not having their sexual health needs met?
- What about those whose bodies are not respected in the sexuality dialogue?

Where are their voices in this movement?

Sex positivity is too often synonymous with "everything about sex must be positive." Sex-positive thought should not assume everyone has the same positive, uncomplicated feelings toward sex. For example, just in the past couple of years we have seen a huge amount of attention being brought to the widespread issue of sexual assault in our country, bringing to light the voices of survivors with the #MeToo campaign started by Tarana Burke in 2006. Bringing awareness to sexual assault issues is a part of the sex positivity movement: it opens up the conversation for survivors, helps them reclaim their power, and hopefully paves the way for a healthier sex culture.

---

38   World Health Organization, *Defining sexual health*, 1.

Sex-positive ideology needs to address the less-than-positive aspects of sexuality and sexual health if it can truly be considered an inclusive movement. It needs to include the issues and the people still rarely talked about, or even known about. Sex being a consistently taboo topic, it may come as no surprise our society likes to shove the more uncomfortable bits under the rug, choosing to remark on "it" using playful euphemisms or crude gestures.

These childish ways of referring to the dreaded "S" word follow us well into adulthood and point to a general lack of appropriate or comprehensive sexual education in our schools. At least in the adult world we are introduced to the pleasurable side of sex. In school, more often than not, the habit is to cherry pick the biggest consequences of sex (hello graphic pictures of sexually transmitted infections and horrifically drawn-out birthing videos) and, quite literally, avoid anything else.

We have a long history of selectivity when it comes to sex ed in this country. Before organized sex ed, information on the topic often came from health reformers distributing pamphlets warning about the "immense evils" of masturbation, which they warned could cause constipation, warts, insanity, and death.[39] The first sex ed classes began to appear in school curriculums in the 1920s, inspired by the military's sex ed programs which warned soldiers of the dangers of diseases such as syphilis.[40] Up until the 1960s, sexual educa-

---

39 *Science and Its Times: Understanding the Social Significance of Scientific Discovery,* s.v. "The Study of Human Sexuality," accessed August 21, 2020.

40 Johannah Cornblatt, "A Brief History of Sex Ed in America," *Newsweek,* October 27, 2009.

tion, faithfully governed by the moral purity activists and the American Social Hygiene Association (ASHA), consisted of preventing STIs, extinguishing the horrors of masturbation and prostitution, and condemning premarital sex.[41]

Quote from an ASHA "Keeping Fit" poster for young males circa 1920: "Somewhere the girl who may become your wife is keeping clean for YOU. YOU EXPECT HER TO REMAIN PURE. Will you take to her a life equally clean?"[42]

Quote from the ASHA pamphlet titled The Case Against the Red Light: "Moreover, when prostitution is easily accessible, men form the habit of seeking it with greater frequency. New girls must fill this demand. The man-about-town finds his appetite for prostitution artificially stimulated by the district and he goes out and creates a new prostitute from some weak-willed and trustful girl. Thus, the red-light district changes normal women into prostitutes."[43]

As support for sex ed in schools began to grow through the 60s and 70s, it seemed as if the country was on track for comprehensive

41 "History of Sex Education in the U.S.," Planned Parenthood, November 2016, 1; John P. Elia, "School-Based Sexuality Education: A Century of Sexual and Social Control," in *Sexuality Education - Past Present and Future*, ed. Elizabeth Schroder and Judy Kuriansky (Westport, CT: Praeger, 2009), 33.

42 Keeping Fit– An Exhibit for Older Boys and Young Men, 10, 1919-1922, Box 171, Folder 8, American Social Health Association Records, University of Minnesota Libraries, Social Welfare History Archives.

43 American Social Hygiene Association, *The Case Against the Red Light* (New York: United States Public Health Service, 1920), 2-3, Box 54, Folder "Social Hygiene," Adèle Goodman Clark papers 1849-1978, VCU Libraries Gallery.

sexual health education.[44] In 1964, Mary Calderone, the medical director for Planned Parenthood, founded the Sexuality Information and Education Council of the United States (SIECUS) with the goal of providing accurate information to young people and adults about sex, sexuality, and sexual health, challenging ASHA's monopoly on sex education curriculum development.[45]

But the sexual revolution of the 60s spurred fierce pushback from religious conservatives opposed to sexual education in public schools.[46] The John Birch Society and the Christian Crusade condemned SIECUS and sex ed for "promoting promiscuity and moral depravity and rumors abounded concerning what instructors were teaching in classes."[47] Some argued sex instructors were stripping, performing sex, and encouraging homosexuality in class, while Gordon Drake and James Hargis argued in their widely distributed pamphlet "Is the School House the Proper Place to Teach Raw Sex?" that sex ed would brainwash America's children with communist ideologies.[48]

> *"If the new morality is affirmed, our children will become easy targets for Marxism and other amoral, nihilistic philosophies—as well as V.D.!"*[49]

44 "History of Sex," Planned Parenthood, 1.
45 "History of Sex," Planned Parenthood, 2; "Our History," SIECUS, accessed August 31, 2020; *Science and Its Times: Understanding the Social Significance of Scientific Discovery*, s.v. "The Study of Human Sexuality," accessed August 21, 2020.
46 *Science and Its Times: Understanding the Social Significance of Scientific Discovery*, s.v. "The Study of Human Sexuality," accessed August 21, 2020.
47 Ibid.
48 Ibid.
49 Ibid.

A return to more conservative values in the 80s also threatened to reverse any progress in the field. A debate erupted between implementing thorough, information-based sex ed versus abstinence-only programs after Congress passed the Adolescent Family Life Act (AFLA) to promote "chastity education." The American Civil Liberties Union (ACLU) later challenged this law in court, claiming it violated the separation of church and state, at the expense of public school children.[50]

The HIV/AIDS pandemic beginning in 1981 pushed formal sex ed instructions for adolescents on topics such as contraception, condoms, and STIs through the mid-1990s. The epidemic also saw the birth of federally financed education materials required to stress sexual abstinence and forbidding information on homosexuality and drug use.[51] Eventually, the "welfare reform" of the late 90s marked the adoption of abstinence-only-until-marriage (AOUM) sex education as the US' singular approach to adolescent sexual health.[52]

Abstinence-only programs are based on the belief exposing youth to "medically accurate, comprehensive information

---

50 "History of Sex," Planned Parenthood, 1, 7; Leslie M. Kantor et al., "Abstinence-only policies and programs: An overview," *Sexuality Research & Social Policy* 5, no.6 (September 2008): 6.

51 "A Timeline of HIV and AIDS," HIV.gov, accessed September 22, 2020; Jill Lawrence, "Senate Says Federal AIDS Education Material Can't Promote Homosexuality," AP News, October 14, 1987.

52 Kelli S. Hall et al., "The State of Sex Education in the United States," *Journal of Adolescent Health* 58, no. 6 (June 2016): 595; Heather D. Boonstra, "Advocates Call for a New Approach After the Era of 'Abstinence-Only' Sex Education," *Guttmacher Policy Review* 12, no. 1 (March 2009): 6-7; John Santelli et al., "Abstinence and abstinence-only education: a review of U.S. policies and programs," *Journal of Adolescent Health* 38, no. 1 (January 2006): 75.

would increase [their] risk-taking behaviors," a theory predicated on fear-mongering and traditional values, with no evidence to support its claim:[53]

Highlights from a 2004 report on thirteen AOUM programs released by Representative Henry Waxman:

- Eleven of the thirteen curricula contained errors and distortions.
- The curricula contained false and misleading information about the effectiveness of contraception, HIV prevention, and condoms.
- The curricula contained false and misleading information about the risks of abortion.
- The curricula blurred religious belief with science.
- The curricula treated stereotypes about girls and boys as scientific fact. The stereotypes:
  - undermine girls' achievements
  - promote the myth that girls are weak and need protection
  - reinforce sexual aggression among men.
- The curricula contained false and misleading information about the risks of sexual activity, including information about cervical cancer prevention, HIV risk behaviors, chlamydia, and mental health.
- The curricula contained scientific errors.[54]

---

53 "History of Sex," Planned Parenthood, 1; Kantor et al., "Abstinence-only," 6.

54 "History of Sex," Planned Parenthood, 8; Henry Waxman, "The Content of Federally Funded Abstinence-Only Programs," United States House of Representatives Committee on Government Reform, December 2004.

Highlights from three additional AOUM evaluations conducted in 2007, all of which found the programs to be ineffective:

- No program helped raise the age of first intercourse.
- No program helped teens postpone having sex.
- No program helped sexually active teens become sexually abstinent.
- No program helped reduce the number of teens' sex partners.
- No program helped improve the use of condoms or other contraceptives among sexually active teens.[55]

Despite extensive research demonstrating AOUM's lack of efficacy in preventing pregnancy, reducing risky behaviors, delaying sexual initiation, or improving sexual health outcomes in any way, abstinence-only programs have received over $2.2 billion worth of funding since the inception of the movement, and continue to remain well-funded to this day.[56] These programs have been used for decades to push ideological messages—often rooted in conservative religious beliefs—promoting damaging gender stereotypes and homophobic sentiments.

---

55   "History of Sex," Planned Parenthood, 9-10; Douglas Kirby, *Emerging Answers 2007: Research Findings on Programs to Reduce Teen Pregnancy and Sexually Transmitted Diseases* (Washington, DC: National Campaign to Prevent Teen and Unplanned Pregnancy, 2007), 102, accessed May 30, 2020; Christopher Trenholm et al., *Impacts of Four Title V, Section 510 Abstinence Education Programs* (Princeton, NJ: Mathematica Policy Research, 2007), 59-61, accessed May 30, 2020; Kristen Underhill, Paul Montgomery, and Don Operario, "Sexual abstinence only programmes to prevent HIV infection in high income countries: systematic review," *BMJ* 335, no. 7613 (August 2007): 1.

56   "History of Sex," Planned Parenthood, 7; "A History of AOUM Funding," SIECUS, 2019.

Establishing strict gender roles and upholding heterosexuality confines adolescents' sexuality to a very narrow path and values the preservation of traditional norms over the healthy psychological development of youth. For girls, AOUM espouses being socially and sexually submissive to men. This strips girls of sexual agency and signals a lack of autonomy to make their own sexual decisions, which can often result in unhealthy and unwanted sexual experiences.[57]

These gender stereotypes can be even more pervasive and harmful to women of color. Studies have shown women in the Latina community, surrounded by *machismo* attitudes, are likely to subscribe to prescriptive roles undermining women's self-determination, like virgin or caretaker. In the Black community, a woman's "respectability" may be thrown into question the more sexual partners she has had.[58]

---

57 Julie F. Kay and Ashley Jackson, *Sex, Lies & Stereotypes: How Abstinence-Only Programs Harm Women and Girls* (New York: Legal Momentum, 2008), 21, accessed May 30, 2020; Janet Holland et al., "Sex, gender and power: young women's sexuality in the shadow of AIDS," *Sociology of Health & Illness* 12, no. 3 (September 1990): 343; Susan L. Davies, "Predictors of Inconsistent Contraceptive Use among Adolescent Girls: Findings from a Prospective Study," *Journal of Adolescent Health* 39, no. 1 (July 2006): 47.

58 Kay, *Sex, Lies,* 22; Stephen T. Russell and Faye C. H. Lee, "Practitioners' Perspectives on Effective Practices for Hispanic Teenage Pregnancy Prevention," *Perspectives on Sexual and Reproductive Health* 36, no. 4 (Summer 2004): 143; Jennifer J. Frost and Anne K. Driscoll, *Sexual and reproductive health of U.S. Latinas: a literature review* (New York: Guttmacher Institute, 2006), 29-30, accessed May 30, 2020; Katherine Andrinopoulos, Deanna Kerrigan, and Jonathan M. Ellen, "Understanding Sex Partner Selection From the Perspective of Inner-City Black Adolescents," *Perspectives on Sexual and Reproductive Health* 38, no. 3 (September 2006): 135; Mindy Thompson Fullilove et al., "Black Women and AIDS Prevention: A View Toward Understanding the Gender Rules," *The Journal of Sex Research* 27, no. 1 (February 1990): 53-54.

***

In general, the sex ed curriculum in the US can be described as a "patchwork" of information and practices, lacking standard teachings and implementation processes resulting in a hodgepodge of biased misinformation, religious ideologies, and mediocre instruction.

As of 2020:

- Only twenty-seven states and DC mandate sex education and HIV education.
- Only seventeen states require such programs be medically accurate.
- Thirty-nine states and DC require provision of information on abstinence, while only twenty (nearly half) require provision of information on contraception.
- Nineteen states require instruction on the importance of engaging in sexual activity *only within marriage.*
- Only ten states and DC require inclusive content with regard to sexual orientation.
- Only nine states require instruction that is appropriate for a student's cultural background and not biased against any race, sex, or ethnicity.

Only eight states require instruction on the importance of consent to sexual activity.[59]

---

59 "Sex and HIV Education," Guttmacher Institute, last modified September 1, 2020.

This means, in the majority of states, the basics of safe sex practices are not a requirement in sex ed, white, hetero, gendered norms propagate, and consensual sex practices are one of the least prioritized topics of adolescent sexual health. After twelve years of schooling, most eighteen-year-olds can confidently tell you the mitochondria is the powerhouse of the cell but balk at the idea of saying the word "vagina."

Failing to appropriately address even the basics of sexual health signals to adolescents sex is a taboo topic.

Additionally, women are particularly under scrutiny when it comes to our sexuality. We still are often viewed through a puritanical lens and we face unique barriers when we do endure sexual health or sexuality issues. Moreover, when sexual education lacks emphasis on healthy, consensual relationships and fails to view sexual expression as an integral part to everyone in the relationship, it woefully under-prepares adolescents entering a sexually inundated world to understand or handle the complexities of sexuality and sexual health.

A failing sex ed system allows for environments like the "hookup culture" to permeate teen and young adult lives, something professor Lisa Wade describes as "an occupying force, coercive and omnipresent."[60] While exciting for some, the idea everyone is and *should* be having sex all the time, casually, with a bunch of different people is a source of anxiety for those who want to opt out but don't feel they can.[61] This isn't the culture sex-positive ideology is trying to build.

---

60 Lisa Wade, *American Hookup: The New Culture of Sex on Campus* (New York: W. W. Norton & Company, 2017), 14.

61 Wade, *American Hookup*, 14-16.

But the messages young people are receiving about healthy sex are so convoluted or so entirely absent that navigating the waters of sexuality, sexual health, and emotional well-being becomes treacherous.

What happens when we construct an environment which simultaneously signals sex as an irresistible social necessity and as something whose inner workings and complications should be pushed to the back burner?

When women are methodically trained to put others' needs above our own, speaking up when something is wrong, especially about a topic we have been told is going to make other people feel uncomfortable, becomes increasingly difficult.

Unsurprisingly, we end up with a significant group of women and assigned female at birth (AFAB) individuals who receive limited sex ed and who are not able to easily fit themselves into the neat little spaces constructed for them. They are left with questions:

Why does everyone else seem to fit seamlessly with these sexual norms?

Why am I left flailing alone?

Why, if sexuality is such a pervasive topic, is no one talking about what I am going through?

The answers lie in the layers upon layers of messages about sex from decades past which continue to rule mainstream sex ed today. It's a story of damaging stereotypes and misinformation which focuses on the experiences and the values of a few, while leaving everyone else out. It's a product of our history which has never fully treated sexual health as a public health issue, but the buried issues of female sexual health do not remain in the past. They are very much still alive in the present and are broadly and consistently ignored.

CHAPTER 2

Unsung Failings of the Medical Community

Squeaky sneakers echo loudly as the girl's high school basketball team sprints across the freshly polished gymnasium floor. As they each reach the other side, they pivot and begin sprinting back. Lara huffs out quick breaths, her long legs carrying her quickly across the gym. Just as she turns to complete her final sprint, she feels a stabbing pain shoot through her abdomen. Much worse than the side stitches she sometimes gets while running, she crumples onto the floor.

"I literally felt like I was dying," she recalls. "My body remembers that pain so vividly."[62]

Her mom rushed Lara to the emergency room as she gasped in agony. As they entered the examination room, Lara set her backpack on the chair next to her mom and sat doubled-over on the examination table, paper crinkling under her legs. She waited for the doctor to ask her questions, to try and

---

62 *As/Is*, "My Doctor Didn't Believe My Pain," September 2, 2017, video, 10:05.

figure out what was wrong. Instead, the doctor's attention was captured by a button pinned to Lara's backpack.

"What's that button for?" she asked.

"Oh, um, it's in memory of my classmate who passed away," Lara replied.

Understanding registered on her doctor's face and she knowingly turned to Lara's mom. "I see what's going on," she concluded, "your daughter is just grieving. It's very common for teens to go through something like this after a tragedy."

She then reached over and plucked the button from the bag before holding it in front of Lara's face. "Now, say goodbye to your friend," she instructed Lara, "Like you mean it."

Confused, Lara turned her attention to the pin and forced out a muddled farewell to her friend. She then turned expectantly back to the doctor, waiting for her to run some tests or prescribe some treatment for her excruciating pain. But the doctor simply smiled and told Lara she should be feeling better shortly. Then she left. She thought she had just cured Lara's problem.

But less than four years later, Lara's invisible pain struck again. This time, she was on the treadmill when it hit so suddenly, she fell on the still-running machine, scuffing her knees before crawling her way to the women's bathroom to throw up. Her friend, overhearing, called an ambulance and got her to the hospital. After waiting hours, she was finally let in to see a doctor.

Back on the examination table, with the same crinkling of paper under her legs, Lara hoped for a real diagnosis or explanation this time. Instead, the doctor simply told her the symptoms were from PMS and to take Advil next time.

The next time it happened, Lara didn't even want to go to the doctor. She was experiencing pain akin to being stabbed over and over, and all she wanted to do was lie in her bed alone and die. She didn't want to go back to see someone who was just going to tell her the pain was all in her head or just normal period pain, not when she still felt so much shame and embarrassment from going the first two times and being told she was imagining or exaggerating her pain.

Years later when she finally was diagnosed with endometriosis and discovered the pain she was experiencing was due to ovarian cysts bursting, she felt vindicated, but also angry. Not only was she made to feel like she was imagining things for years and felt forced to bury her pain rather than seek medical help, she had to live without a diagnosis or any treatment because her doctors refused to believe her.[63]

> *Endometriosis is a disorder in which the tissue which normally lines the inside of the uterus begins to grow outside the uterus, spreading to the other pelvic organs. Since this tissue acts as endometrial tissue would, it thickens, breaks down, and bleeds with each menstrual cycle. As it has no way to exit the body, it becomes trapped, potentially forming cysts in the ovaries and lesions in the surrounding tissue.[64]*

---

63 Ibid.
64 "Endometriosis," Mayo Clinic, accessed September 1, 2020.

Doctors not believing women's pain and women not receiving proper treatment is so common there are too many examples to count. Studies have shown women's pain is more likely than men's to be attributed as "psychosomatic," or a product of emotional distress, and therefore often undervalued and misdiagnosed. According to a National Pain Report survey, out of 2,400 women with chronic pain issues, 90 percent reported experiencing gender discrimination in the health care system from their providers.[65]

"I can't tell you how many women I've seen who have gone to see numerous doctors, only to be told their issues were stress-related or all in their heads," says Dr. Fiona Gupta, a neurologist and movement disorders specialist in the department of neurosurgery at the Icahn School of Medicine at Mount Sinai in New York City. "They knew something was wrong but had been discounted and instructed not to trust their own intuition."[66]

***

In 2015, Jessica, a young, healthy twenty-something-year-old was having the time of her life. Living in New York City, working at her dream job, she was ready to take on the post-grad world. That is, until her body decided to rudely interrupt her sex life.

65 Camille Noe Pagán, "When Doctors Downplay Women's Health Concerns," *New York Times*, May 3, 2018; Pat Anson, "Women in Pain Report Significant Gender Bias," National Pain Report, September 12, 2014.

66 Pagán, "When Doctors."

"I started to develop pain," she recalls, her voice noticeably dropping as she finishes with, "in my vagina."[67]

She began noticing it mostly during sex, an uncomfortable burning sensation, which gradually grew in intensity over the coming months. Naturally, she made an appointment with her gynecologist and showed up for her examination later that week. In her doctor's office, she explained the issues she had been having and expressed her suspicion that something was wrong.

"I just want to know if you think something looks off or abnormal."

In response, her doctor flat out laughed at her. No treatment, no referrals, not even an acknowledgment of her concerns. She was laughed at, assured she was fine, and told to go home. Wondering if she was just making a big deal out of nothing, and ashamed for bringing it up at all, she decided to simply ignore the issue.

Resolving to abstain from any sexual activity for the time being, she hoped the pain would vanish on its own. Instead, her symptoms only worsened over the next year. She saw four other doctors during that time, jumping from one to the next as each one failed to help. Two more told her nothing was wrong with her. A third treated her for herpes, and when that did nothing to alleviate her symptoms, the doctor backtracked and told her nothing was wrong with her. A

---

67   *As/Is,* "My Doctor."

fourth was convinced Jessica's pain was all in her head and wanted to put her on antidepressants.

Throughout all of her doctor's visits, her pain was never truly validated, and she was never offered a diagnosis or even a referral to see someone who might have more expertise and knowledge about her condition. In terms of information, she was presented with some vague pamphlets about women's health. She tried doing her own research, but without proper medical guidance or explanation, she was still unclear about her condition and how to proceed.[68]

Not that it should have been her responsibility to diagnose and treat herself.

Imagine if a patient came in complaining of a rash on their arm that appeared a week ago and was itching and burning and clearly causing them discomfort. Instead of the doctor asking the patient questions about their medical history and their symptoms or running tests, and then prescribing medication based on their professional findings, they laughed and said, "I don't think anything's wrong with you. But if you are really convinced, here are some pamphlets on rashes. Maybe those will help you figure out what's wrong."

It's antithetical to think a doctor would shame a patient for their condition, and not offer medical help or advice to someone experiencing pain or discomfort just because the pain is not visible, they don't believe the patient, or they're unfamiliar with the patient's condition.

---

68 Ibid.

Women's pain is too often minimized by many in the health care community. The medical education system in the US is leaving a huge gap in the area of female sexual health, to the point gynecologists don't know how to diagnosis, treat, or refer patients with vaginal pain because the subject is under-researched and rarely emphasized as an important concern for female sexual health.[69]

"There's not really a lot of information about the vagina," Jessica comments. "What I learned from my own research is there's just blanket terms. Vestibulina, vestibulitis, vulvadina, and they're all just blanket terms for: 'There's pain in different parts of your vagina.' But there's no cure. The pamphlets say, 'Use lube!' or 'Try to think of something else other than sex!'"[70]

This is especially concerning when doctors turning a blind eye to females' pain becomes a life or death issue.

Les Henderson is one such case, in which her doctors' consistent tendency to ignore her pain eventually landed her in the hospital. Around the age of ten or eleven, when she started her period, Les began to experience intense abdominal pain every month.

"Probably just bad period cramps," said her mom and grandma.

"Nothing to worry about," said her doctor.

---

69 Nicola Slawson, "'Women have been woefully neglected': does medical science have a gender problem?" The Guardian, December 18, 2019.
70 *As/Is*, "My Doctor."

As her symptoms followed her into adulthood, she continued to seek medical advice, wherein she was often accused of fabricating or inflating her pain. That is until she spent a week in the hospital due to a collapsed lung.

It was 2016 and a huge snowstorm had just blown in. Les had been staying in a hotel down in Navy Yard, DC for a work conference, and she rose early the morning before her first session with a hankering for some coffee and an egg mcmuffin. Stretching, she spotted a McDonald's through her window across the street.

Swinging her legs out of bed, she felt her chest constrict as she stood, like a bag of bricks had been placed on her chest and her lungs couldn't fill properly. Shaking her head to clear the white flashes beginning to appear in her vision, Les figured she stood up too fast. Steadying herself, she bundled up and headed into the chilly morning air.

Crunching through the snow, Les reached the McDonald's out of breath, feeling as if she had just run a marathon after walking barely two blocks. Throughout the rest of the day, she felt like she couldn't catch her breath, and finally decided to go to an urgent care clinic that night. She thought maybe she was just overstressed, or needed to reevaluate her diet, and they could just give her some medicine and she could leave.

But when she got to the clinic and they took some x-rays they found her lung 80 percent collapsed.

Suddenly, everything and everyone burst into action. Les was strapped to a gurney and rushed into an ambulance to take her to the hospital. She called her partner from the ambulance crying hysterically. She didn't know what was going on, no one would tell her anything. When she got to the hospital, nurses and EMTs started shouting:

"We've got a patient, her lung's collapsed!"

"It's her right lung, her right lung is 80 percent collapsed!"

"How long? We don't know how long."

"She's not breathing properly!"

A hospital worker appeared at Les' side as she was briskly wheeled down the corridor and started rapid firing questions:

"Do you smoke? Did you have too many hits off a bong? How many blunts have you smoked in the last day?"

"No, no, no," Less managed to rasp out, "I don't know how this happened."

Then they stuck a tube into her chest to help with her breathing and told her she needed surgery, so she could only have liquids for the next twelve hours. They ended up postponing the surgery for several days, reducing Les to a scared, frustrated, hungry mess by the time of her procedure.

On top of that, there was something wrong with her breathing tube. It felt like it had shifted and was now choking her.

"I think there's something wrong with my chest tube," she told her nurse, "Can you wheel me to radiology?"

"There's nothing wrong with your chest tube. You're fine," was the response.

"Really, I can't breathe. Can you take me to radiology?" Les tried again.

"She's hysterical," her nurse spoke over her head to a younger nurse, "Give her a Xanax."

"I don't need a goddamn Xanax; I need to go to radiology!" Les screamed.

After a startled pause and with eyebrows raised, the nurses finally acceded. As they wheeled her to radiology, Les' breaths came in spasms as she struggled to suck in oxygen. Sure enough, they found the chest tube had shifted onto Les' windpipe, blocking her airflow.

Moreover, when they finally proceeded with Les' surgery, they discovered she had a rare and particularly dangerous case of endometriosis.

In most cases, endometriosis will involve the ovaries, fallopian tubes, and the tissue lining your pelvis. In rare cases, the tissue will grow past the pelvic organs.[71] In Les' body, they found the tissue growing outside her uterus had spread past the pelvic area to reach all the way to her lungs.

Luckily, her surgery was successful and Les recovered from the traumatic experience. But the question remains:

---

71 "Endometriosis," Mayo Clinic.

If her condition was so severe, severe enough to land her in the hospital, how did it escape multiple doctors for years?

Why, even when she was in the hospital with a severely collapsed lung, was she still not taken seriously?

While women of all backgrounds face the stigma of not being believed by their healthcare providers, there is no doubt that the medical system is biased against people of color, the LGBTQ+ community, and lower income individuals and their families. Les, a black, working-class, lesbian woman, was most likely a victim of these systemic faults, on top of the fact she was dealing with an "invisible" illness that made it exponentially easier for doctors to ignore.

Implicit bias, attitudes that lie outside of conscious awareness, are alive and well in the medical system. Similar to the general US public, health care providers hold unconscious biases toward racial minorities, which can ultimately lead to harmful judgments and improper treatment.

In fact, a systematic review of fifteen studies found most health care providers have implicit positive attitudes toward whites and negative attitudes toward people of color.[72] According to Dayna Bowen Matthew, a professor of law at the University of Virginia School of Law, these biases, which physicians are likely unaware of, help to explain racial disparities in health care. As a result, patient-provider interactions

---

72 William J. Hall et al., "Implicit Racial/Ethnic Bias Among Health Care Professionals and Its Influence on Health Care Outcomes: A Systematic Review," *American Journal of Public Health* 105, no. 12 (December 2015): 60.

involving people of color are often characterized by, "dominant communication styles, fewer demonstrated positive emotions, infrequent requests for input about treatment decisions, and less patient-centered care."[73]

Repeated instances of provider bias will then diminish trust between patients and their provider, which can dissuade people of color to seek help or to speak candidly with their physician in the future.

On the other end, repeated cases of specific patient behavior may solidify the biases providers already hold until they become fixed "truths" for the whole group.

According to a study conducted by the National Institute of Health, it eventually becomes easier to lump a person into an established set of characteristics for their racial group than to treat the person as an individual with unique characteristics independent of any stereotypes of their group.[74] Building genuine relationships with their patients to administer equitable, personalized, and beneficial treatment is difficult to do when the doctor fails to truly listen to and see their patient in favor of making generalized assumptions.

Unsurprisingly, women of color's pain gets ignored more often than white women's, to the point of serious health consequences. For example, no one knows this better than pregnant women of color who face severe health complications because of health providers' assumptions of incompetence.

---

73 Khlara M. Bridges, "Implicit Bias and Racial Disparities in Health Care," American Bar Association, accessed April 26, 2020.

74 William J. Hall et al., "Implicit Racial/Ethnic Bias," 61.

Just two years ago two high profile celebrities, Serena Williams and Beyoncé, faced life-threatening complications in their respective pregnancies, alerting the public to how pervasive prejudice in the medical field can be and exposing some of the worst consequences negligence and implicit biases produce.[75]

***

Tressie was four months pregnant when the bleeding started one day at work.

"When you are black woman, having a body is already complicated for workplace politics," she says, "having a bleeding, distended body is especially egregious."[76]

Apparently, that remains true even at an obstetrics office. Upon arriving at the clinic, she sat in the waiting room for a half hour, despite calling ahead and explaining her condition when she checked in. She quickly bled through the waiting room chair, much to the disgust of the nurse assigned to collect her, before finally being granted access to a private room. Her doctor then downplayed her concerns and told her spotting was normal before sending her home.

Later that night, she began to feel cramping in her glutes. After trying to walk it off, stretch it out, and relax in a hot bath, she finally called the nurse.

---

75 "Why are black women at such high risk of dying from pregnancy complications?" American Heart Association News, February 20, 2019.

76 Tressie McMillan Cottom, *Thick: And Other Essays* (New York: The New Press, 2019), 75.

"Hi, I was in earlier today because I was bleeding. I'm now experiencing some pain in my glutes."

"Okay, and does your back hurt?"

"No, my ass hurts. It's been cramping for hours."

"Alright, it's probably just constipation. Try to go to the bathroom."

So, Tressie tried that for the next three days, but after not sleeping for more than fifteen consecutive minutes in seventy-two hours, she decided it was time to go to the hospital. At the hospital, consumption of bad food was offered as a possibility for her symptoms.

Eventually they did an ultrasound and found her child surrounded by two tumors, each larger than the baby itself.

The doctor turned and offhandedly remarked, "If you make it through the night without going into preterm labor, I'd be surprised," and then left. As the nurse wheeled her to the maternity ward, she revealed Tressie had been in labor for the past three days.

"You should have said something!" she chided Tressie.

The next few hours were a haze of pain and stress as Tressie slipped in and out of consciousness, meeting unfriendly and begrudgingly cooperative faces each time she surfaced. She remembers waking up as she pushed out her tiny daughter, who died just minutes later. Exhausted and emotionally drained, cradling her dead daughter, the only words of "comfort" she received came from her nurse:

"Just so you know, there was nothing we could have done, because you didn't tell us you were in labor."

Tressie recognizes the system churning out medical professionals is biased against her and other black women, viewing them as incompetent—ignorant of their own bodies.

"All of my status characteristics screamed 'competent,' but nothing could shut down what my blackness screams when I walk into the room...what does that say about how poorer, average black women are treated?"[77]

Pregnancy complications and their consequences are certainly one of the worst-case scenarios with doctor negligence. As one of the richest countries in the world, the US has the worst maternal mortality rate in any industrialized country and suffers from black women perishing in childbirth at rates similar to those in developing nations.[78] According to the Centers for Disease Control and Prevention, Black, American Indian, and Alaska Native (AI/AN) women die from pregnancy-related issues at two to three times the rate of white women.[79]

---

77 McMillan Cottom, *Thick*, 80, 82.

78 McMillan Cottom, *Thick*, 79, 80; Nicholas J. Kassebaum et al., "Global, regional, and national levels of maternal mortality, 1990–2015: a systematic analysis for the Global Burden of Disease Study 2015," *Lancet* 388, 10053 (October 2016): 1784.

79 Emily E. Petersen et al., "Racial/Ethnic Disparities in Pregnancy-Related Deaths — United States, 2007–2016," *Morbidity and Mortality Weekly Report* 68, no. 35 (September 2019): 762.

"Pain, like pregnancy, is inconvenient for bureaucratic efficiency and has little use in a capitalist regime," says Tressie. "When the medical profession systematically denies the existence of black women's pain, underdiagnoses our pain, refuses to alleviate or treat our pain, health care marks us as incompetent bureaucratic subjects. Then it serves us accordingly."[80]

All this begs the question: *Why is this so worrying in the context of sexual health?*

Health care providers invalidating women's health concerns, and further invalidating women of color, disempowers these patients to advocate for themselves and express concern over a sensitive subject already not talked about openly or shrouded in euphemisms.

"As women, we've been taught from an early age to rationalize warning signs of physical or mental health problems," says Dr. Gupta.[81]

Women are conditioned and expected to be polite, to avoid being overly dramatic, to not take up space; it comes to a point where we begin to minimize our own health in favor of adhering to this internalized mold.

Further, health care providers who then repeatedly fail to value women's concerns exacerbate the power imbalance and position women at an additional disadvantage. It is important

---

80 McMillan Cottom, *Thick*, 79.
81 Pagán, "When Doctors."

to recognize there is a difference between self-diagnosing and recognizing your pain or condition is not being taken seriously or being properly understood by your practitioner. It is also important to recognize you are not overreacting or being neurotic.

Dr. Gupta advises, "If you feel like something isn't right with your health, honor that—even if a doctor is disagreeing with you. It's better to find out you're wrong than to wait too long."[82]

Unsurprisingly, our long history of suppressing female sexuality and failing to prioritize female sexual health issues in mainstream sexual education has firmly cemented itself within the sterile white walls of our hospitals and utilitarian white coats of our physicians. There are so many stories of doctors dismissing valid concerns from women and AFAB individuals that I'm beginning to wonder if it's their part-time hobby.

As we'll see in later chapters, this phenomenon of not believing women or not appropriately addressing and legitimizing their issues cycles into declining emotional health, self-image, and sense of sexuality, further hindering female sexual liberation.

---

82 Ibid.

CHAPTER 3

A Preview

In the following chapters, we'll take a deeper look at some commonly ignored, undervalued, and misunderstood sexual health issues affecting millions of women and AFAB individuals in the US every day. Through anecdotal and expert testimonies, we'll gain a clearer understanding of how certain problems and groups of people are pushed under the rug and made "invisible" from a lack of awareness or convenience on the part of the general public and medical community, and the negative impacts stemming from this invalidation.

Part two of the book begins with an exploration of often overlooked physical vaginal and vulvar pain issues. Chapter four focuses on vaginismus and endometriosis and Chapter five delves into vulvodynia. For each issue, we look at both the physical symptoms and effects, as well as the mental impacts and strain on one's sense of sexuality.

Chapters six and seven take a look at an issue which straddles the line between sexual health and mental health. Premenstrual dysphoric disorder (PMDD), often confused with the more widely known premenstrual syndrome (PMS), is a salient example of a period problem which regularly goes unchecked and untreated for years. These two chapters demonstrate how societal tendencies to generalize period symptoms and normalize PMS can have life-threatening consequences.

Chapters eight and nine explore the intersection of sexuality and disability. In these chapters, we'll analyze how certain stereotypes about people with disabilities impacts their relationship with their sexuality and bars them from the sexuality conversation. We also look at the improvements needed in sexual health care to ensure medical inclusivity for women with disabilities.

Chapter ten delves into transgender and nonbinary sexuality and sexual health issues. We'll examine how tendencies to delegitimize people with vaginas in the medical field is exacerbated for people who do not present or identify as typically female. We'll also look at how inadequate training and information on trans health leaves medical practitioners incapable of appropriately addressing trans peoples' specific needs. Finally, we'll see how societal stigmas and a lack of protective laws can threaten non-cis identifying people's freedom of sexual expression.

Part two concludes with Chapter eleven, which examines the prevalence of female genital mutilation in the US. We will analyze why this human rights violation continues in our country, and the physical and emotional trauma it induces.

Part three explores the importance and benefits of more comprehensive and understanding of sexual health care in the medical arena. Chapter twelve addresses the implications of layered vulnerabilities within female sexual health and sexuality, and the need to consider individual barriers and concerns in the context of multiple systemic factors.

Chapter thirteen looks at the benefits of specialized women's sexual health care in appropriately treating the physical pain issues standard medical care may miss or treat incorrectly.

Finally, Chapter fourteen discusses how general practitioners and OB/GYNs can better serve a range of patients and issues. This chapter looks at the importance of education specifically on female pain, disparities in menstrual cycles, different sexualities, and so on, in providing the most inclusive care possible, and lessons to extend to sex ed in schools for the general public.

PART 2

OPENING
THE TRAP

CHAPTER 4

All Pain, No Gain?

"How was it? Did it hurt?" are the first questions out of any female friends mouth after their girlfriend's "first time."

"Ugh, I'm sorry. How are your cramps? Do you need any Advil?" are the immediate responses after learning your friend has just started her period.

These automatic reactions come from years of messages from parents, doctors, teachers, and peers, that pain during periods and pain during sex—pain with anything surrounding your vagina—is inevitable. In fact, pain is so normalized with women's sexual health that we begin to ignore, disregard, or completely silence legitimate medical issues.

Over the past couple of years, more and more women are coming out to speak their truths about the sometimes-daily pain they have to deal with. About six years ago, Lara Parker, a popular Buzzfeed editor, began publicly documenting her struggles with a slew of "vagina problems," including endometriosis, vaginismus, vulvodynia, and pelvic floor dysfunction.

She amassed quite a following, garnering millions of views on her videos about vaginal Botox, laser therapy, and CBD period products, and is hopeful sharing her story will let others know it is okay, even beneficial, to talk about their pain and it does not make her or them any less of a woman.

For many struggling with these types of issues, however, even acknowledging you experience them or need treatment can be extremely difficult. For one young woman, Savannah, just thinking about her condition only serves to amplify her anxiety.

February of Savannah's freshman year of college, the big moment arrived: she was going to have sex for the first time. We tend to place a lot of emphasis on this so-called "rite of passage" in our society. We want to make sure it's with the right person, at the right time, in the right place.

For Savannah, this was spring semester with one of her friend's fraternity brothers in his dorm room. She had built up the moment in her head for weeks, having to reschedule several times. When the day finally arrived, her nerves were buzzing. She was ready, it was consensual, he was receptive to her needs, but all she felt was pain.

First try—pain.

Second try—pain.

Third try—pain.

A ripping, searing, burning pain which felt as if she were being ripped apart. She tried to ignore it, to push through, to not think about the unendurable pain. But finally, they had to stop trying.

Afterwards, though she physically recovered, feelings of frustration and confusion lingered. She had heard from all of her female friends it hurt when they lost their virginity—*that pain was to be expected.* But as the months wore on, her feelings often shifted toward anxiety when she would think about having sex in any capacity.

I don't understand—how can other women put up with that kind of pain?

Maybe it was the guy. Should I just try again?

Is there something actually wrong with me?

Why can't my body just work like it's supposed to?

As Savannah's frustration mounted, she looked to the internet for answers and discovered she might have some type of pelvic floor dysfunction. However, instead of turning to a medical professional for help, she decided to ignore any potential issues for the time being.

Luckily, Savannah's mother was looking out for her daughter's health and scheduled her first general checkup gynecological exam the summer following her freshman year. At the time, Savannah was nineteen and agreed she should go. She wanted to explore all her birth control options and discuss if getting an IUD was a possibility.

"Ya, I was nervous for sure," she recalls, "but I really thought my OB/GYN would have all the answers and everything would be solved after my appointment."

At the office, with her legs up in the stirrups, Savannah began to feel the obtrusive burning pain rippling up her abdomen as the doctor began her exam. A few excruciating moments later, the doctor, noticing her obvious discomfort, tenderly removed the speculum.

"Sorry," her doctor soothed, "was that hurting you a lot?"

Exhaling, Savannah nodded.

"It seemed as if your muscles were clenching up a lot with the speculum, which was probably causing your pain," her doctor explained. "I think you may have vaginismus, meaning your inner vaginal muscles are involuntarily tensing to the point of pain whenever they come into contact with anything. You may want to try physical therapy; it's been found to be very helpful for people with your condition and..."

As the doctor continued, Savannah nodded along weakly. She wasn't shocked as much as she was disappointed. She had been expecting this sort of diagnosis, and her doctor had just confirmed her fears.

Savannah didn't realize how lucky she was, all things considered, to receive such a prompt diagnosis from a doctor well-versed in vaginal pain conditions. Even so, having her pain validated did little to alleviate the frustration, anxiety, and isolation she felt.

These feelings of frustration and isolation are common among sufferers of vaginismus.

> *"Vaginismus is a psychosexual condition involving the brain subconsciously protecting the vagina from penetration by causing the Kegel muscles to spasm or close. This can cause penetration to be impossible or painful."*[83]

The condition can disrupt or completely obstruct an individual's sex life, and while sometimes the cause can be pinpointed to a specific traumatic event such as a difficult childbirth or sexual abuse, it's often not clear why the vaginal muscles contract.[84] Other common causes include:

- an unpleasant sexual experience or sexual abuse at a young age
- feelings of guilt or shame around sex
- feeling that sexual desire is wrong
- a fear of getting pregnant
- a painful sexual examination
- and experiencing past pain during sexual intercourse, known as dyspareunia, due to:
  - a previous surgery
  - infection of the genital area
  - vaginal dryness
  - and a lack of sexual arousal.[85]

These multiple, and sometimes overlapping, factors can lead an individual to view all or most sexual experiences as painful and to develop a fear of painful sex. As a result, sufferers experience tightened muscles in response to attempted

---

83 "The Vaginismus Network's Guide to Smear Tests," Vaginismus Network, accessed October 2, 2020.

84 "Vaginismus," Health Service Executive, accessed June 15, 2020.

85 Ibid.

penetration, possible burning or stinging pain, and intense fear of penetration. As the body correlates penetration with pain, the vaginal muscles will clench in anticipation as a protective reaction.[86]

Some sufferers of vaginismus describe penetration, whether during sex, during an exam, with a tampon, and so on, as feeling like there's a wall someone is trying to break through, like trying to ram a star-shaped peg into a tiny, round hole, or like someone is ripping them apart with knives from the inside out.[87]

Unsurprisingly, vaginismus can cause emotional distress and relationship issues, especially for sufferers who experience tightening consistently or every time. Addressing the issue requires the individual to work continually, both physically and mentally, on their condition, an often taxing and painful process. Moreover, because it's an uncomfortable topic, it can be embarrassing to talk about, whether with family or even health care providers.

In Savannah's case, she has been reticent to seek further medical help, and though she has found limited comfort from sharing her struggles with a few friends, her parents remain unaware.

Raised an only child in a liberal pocket of North Carolina, Savannah fostered a strong bond with her parents, especially with her mother. That bond continues strong today.

---

86 Ibid.

87 Erin Moynihan, "I Have Vaginismus And It Has Sex So Painful It Feels Like 'Shark Week' In My Vagina," Huffpost, accessed October 2, 2020.

"She's someone I can speak my mind to, we like all the same TV shows, and sometimes she calls me just to hear my voice."

But despite their candor and solid, loving relationship, Savannah is reluctant to reveal her condition to her mother even years later.

"I don't think I have ever really talked to her about my own sexual experiences," she confesses, "it just feels awkward and weird...it's one of those things where I've talked to her about pretty much everything, like drinking and everything, but not sex. The thing is, my mom absolutely would be open to listening about this, it's really more about me because it's embarrassing. And I'm nervous because I feel like if I talk to her about it, it makes it so much more real."

That is, of course, a concern for many people who suffer from vaginismus. *Coming to terms with the diagnosis can feel like you are admitting you are broken in some way.*

Not only is it uncomfortable to talk about, but the journey to recovery is often long, unpleasant, and, in some cases, triggering. As Buzzfeed editor Lara Parker puts it:

"Being told that your vagina doesn't work properly is a scary feeling."[88]

Contrary to Savannah's case, though, Lara went years before her pain was diagnosed as something more than

---

88   Lara Parker, "Learning To Love Life Without Sex," Buzzfeed, April 24, 2014.

psychosomatic, and years more to actually get a complete diagnosis with a constructive course of treatment.

∗∗∗

During Lara's first visit to the gynecologist at the age of thirteen, she sat in the waiting room nervously imagining the uncomfortable stirrups and cold metal speculum she'd heard about and seen on TV. Her mom sat next to her and offered words of encouragement, promising it wouldn't be that bad.

Understandably, Lara was confused when later, lying on the examination table, the speculum betrayed her, inciting an explosion of fiery pain straight through to her abdomen.

She recalls gasping in shock, wondering how, "every woman could just casually tolerate something so excruciating once a year."[89]

Yet, it never occurred to her to ask if maybe her pain wasn't what everyone else experienced. After all, a gynecological exam is a medical service, provided by a professional and is part of most women's regular health care regimen; it's not supposed to provoke pain to the point of being unbearable. *Imagine fearing your body is so defective you can't even handle a normal health checkup.*

Easier to ignore and pretend this is "normal," thought Lara.

She would leave the gynecologist every time in tears. She would feel physically nauseous at the prospect of using a

---

89   Ibid.

tampon. She tried to push through the pain of intercourse, even as it felt as if her insides were tearing apart. After her second failed attempt with intercourse, she made an appointment with her gynecologist that same week. Lying on the same table in the same office, her doctor finally offered up a possible explanation, diagnosing Lara with probable endometriosis.[90]

Possible cysts, scar tissue, and adhesions, common developments from endometriosis, could explain Lara's pain during intercourse, as the endometrial tissue can be pulled and stretched during sex.[91] Her doctor recommended laparoscopic surgery to confirm the diagnosis and remove any visible endometriosis implants and scar tissue.

> *Laparoscopic surgery is a common treatment option for endometriosis, and the only way to diagnose the condition with certainty. During the procedure, a surgeon inserts a viewing instrument through a small incision in the navel and cuts away endometrial tissue to remove any possible cysts or lesions.[92]*

The surgery was scheduled, and Lara returned ready to have her stomach sliced open and her problems solved. They found

---

90 Ibid.

91 Joana Cavaco Silva, "How to prevent endometriosis pain during sex," Medical News Today, April 6, 2018.

92 "Laparoscopic Surgery for Endometriosis," University of Michigan, Michigan Medicine, last modified November 7, 2019.

and removed all the lesions they could, confirming her doctor's diagnosis.[93]

"You're all set," they told her. "You should start feeling better very soon."

A couple weeks later, and Lara was worse than ever.

"It was hardly a miracle cure," she scoffs. "As the weeks went by, I felt continually worse. The pain had not subsided in the least. In fact, it seemed to have heightened."[94]

Her physical pain, with no outlet or release, began to emerge as emotional pain. Shame, embarrassment, and the inevitable physical affliction that came with intimacy eventually caused Lara to give up on that part of her life all together.

She was tired of hearing, *"I don't understand what's wrong with you,"* and not having an answer herself.

She was tired of shying away from any physical touch because it elicited anxiety.

She was tired of trying, when every time her body let her down.

"My 'sexual experience' consisted of doctors poking and prodding me and men looking disappointed at me for something I couldn't explain or help. My doctors told

---

93   Parker, "Learning To Love."
94   Ibid.

me I could have a sexual experience in other ways. But I never bothered to ask them how that would work when I flinched at the mere touch of a man. *They told me there was more to relationships than just sex. I figured that was pretty easy to say when you were able to have sex.*"[95]

Little by little depression began to set in, and her anxiety mounted as college graduation loomed. The idea of starting a full-time job, when some days her pain rendered her immobile and physically shackled her to the couch, terrified her. If nothing else, she needed answers about what was going on with her body.

***

You might not expect one of the top-rated health care systems in the world to be found in small, rural Rochester, Minnesota, but the Mayo Clinic has certainly established a world-renowned reputation since its founding more than a century ago.

The clinic prides itself as being, "a referral center for advanced and complex cases," which is precisely why Lara turned to them in a desperate attempt to find answers.[96] Just after graduation, Lara and her mom hopped in the car, and twelve hours later arrived at the place that would—Lara hoped— offer her some long-awaited relief.

---

95   Lara Parker, "What It's Like To Date When You Can't Have Sex," Buzzfeed News, November 15, 2015.

96   "How the Mayo Clinic Built Its Reputation as a Top Hospital," University of Pennsylvania, August 28, 2018.

Back in the dreaded stirrups, Lara was poked and prodded and poked some more. She tried to find anything to distract herself—squinting so a spot on the wall turned into a pear, listening to the sound of the doctor's wheel-y stool rolling across the linoleum, counting the Q-tips in the glass jar on the counter. She had just gotten to thirty-six when the doctor plucked one from the container to use as a swab in her "next phase of torture."[97]

Suddenly, Lara felt the familiar burning sensation shoot up her abdomen, like a fiery spear stabbing her insides over and over. She yelped at the shock and the doctor removed the Q-tip.

Scrunching her face, the doctor peeled off her gloves.

"Well, it looks like you have a case of vulvodynia and vaginismus." As Lara's face registered confusion, the doctor continued, "You also have some pelvic floor tension myalgia. These are conditions that cause chronic pain in your vagina. Your inner muscles clench up at the slightest touch and cause some pretty extreme pain from the looks of it."

"I don't understand," Lara asked, on the verge of tears. "How did this happen?"

"We don't know. The specific cause of these conditions, and the cures, are not definitive. Unfortunately, I can't tell you that you will ever be completely free of this."

---

97 Parker, "What It's Like."

The tears fell freely now. These weren't the answers Lara was looking for. In fact, they really weren't even answers.

Am I just supposed to live like this for the rest of my life?

She felt nauseous imagining the pain-filled life ahead of her. "Was I supposed to just be okay with the fact they didn't have a fucking cure for it?"[98]

It would have been easy at this moment, as the hope she so viciously clung to dissipated with the doctor's torturous final words, for Lara to give up. Easy for her to let herself believe not only was she broken, but she was unfixable. Her body not a vessel of purpose, protection, and pleasure, but instead a constant betrayal.

Giving into the pain and letting it control her life was never an option for Lara, though. There may not be a definitive cure for her many ailments, but that didn't mean there weren't resources and channels of relief she could draw on to escape the daily constraints her body places on her life.

After the doctor left and Lara's tears dried up, she pushed herself up, wiped her eyes, straightened her ponytail, and decided to keep trying.

That was over six years ago, and since then her road to rehabilitation has not been easy, and she still doesn't know if it will ever be over. But since her visit to the Mayo Clinic, she has refused to remain quiet about her issues any longer. She

---

98 Ibid.

has been writing stories, posting videos, and making meme compilations about her vagina problems and her journey to find relief for years now at Buzzfeed, as well as posting updates (the good, the bad, and the ugly) on her personal social media.

She is in pain, and she wants people to know. But it's not easy for her to reveal this side of her life because her low days are really low, and she would just as soon as forget them than share them for the world to see.

"While I love the idea of raising awareness about endometriosis and other chronic conditions, I've learned I hate sharing these parts of my life because it forces me to relive them," she says.[99]

Weighed down with the baggage—both physical and emotional—of her diagnoses, talking about her ordeals doesn't always lighten the load. Yet Lara is lightening others' loads with her stories. She is helping to spark the discussion and normalize these often ignored and invisible issues. She is using her far-reaching platform and remarkable candor to connect with others who are lost or isolated or hopeless.

"I will continue to try and convince every woman or man that if they're struggling with something like this, they are not alone, and they are not broken."[100]

---

99   Lara Parker, "I Stopped Lying About How Happy I Was On Instagram And Started Telling The Truth About Chronic Pain," Buzzfeed, March 7, 2016.
100 Parker, "Learning To Love."

Broken, incomplete, not a full woman. *For how can you be a full woman if you can't do what every other "normal" woman can do?* "Normal" women can have casual sex, or easily put a tampon in during their period, or go on dates without worrying about when they have to tell the guy sitting across from them their body doesn't "work properly."

These were the things Lara so fiercely wanted to do and be. Or thought she did. She eventually realized, after years of self-loathing and self-pity and self-destructive thoughts, she was trying to fit her body and her life into a box which just wouldn't hold her. Her unique, beautiful self was slowly being chipped away and her self-worth constantly put into question, reinforced by societal norms and her own self-image.

It wasn't until she allowed herself to open up to trusted friends and confidants and allowed herself to be loved as an already complete, full woman that she realized she wasn't broken until she started breaking herself. "I thought I wanted to be able to have pain-free sex. But what I needed was to feel accepted for the way that I am."[101]

***

In recent years, the research and available information on issues like endometriosis and vaginismus has bloomed. There are blogs and Facebook support groups and websites like Endometriosis.net and thevaginismusnetwork.com

---

101 Parker, "What It's Like."

dedicated entirely to informing and building community around these issues. With the internet and social media, it's becoming easier for sufferers to research their conditions and find others like them. Oftentimes, this only helps when they already know what they're looking for.

Without doctors, therapists, and educators pointing them in the right direction, or failing to recognize these issues even exist, sufferers may spend years in the dark or looking in the wrong places.

While getting a confirmed diagnosis is the first step, and a base standard many doctors are still not meeting, effective treatment is the ultimate goal. For endometriosis, there is currently no cure, but there are treatment options intended to relieve symptoms, including medications and surgery. Common medications include:

- NSAIDS (non-steroidal anti-inflammatory drug), which target generalized pain, headaches, and inflammation
- and hormone therapies, like combination or progesterone-only contraceptives and Gn-RH agonists and antagonists, which alter the levels of specific hormones in the body.[102]

High levels of hormones during ovulation, such as estrogen and progesterone, can potentially lead to the growth of endometriosis lesions. So, by suppressing ovarian function and stabilizing hormone levels, the lesions and pain may be reduced.[103]

---

102 "How is Endometriosis Treated?" Endometriosis.net, July 5, 2018.
103 Ibid.

If pain medications and hormone therapy do not work to alleviate symptoms, surgical interventions may be the next step. Surgery is never the first treatment option, though, as the procedure is risky and does not act as a cure.

> *An estimated 20 percent of sufferers who have laparoscopic endometriosis surgery experience the resurgence of symptoms within two years, and 40 percent within five years.*[104]

However, the only way to confirm a diagnosis of endometriosis currently is through laparoscopy.[105] This means a misdiagnosis of endometriosis can lead to an unnecessary surgery, as was the case for Fiona, who we'll meet in the next chapter.

> *Following laparoscopic surgery, some women may choose to have a hysterectomy (removal of the uterus) or a procedure aimed at destroying nerve fibers in the pelvis to reduce pain perception, known as laparoscopic uterine nerve ablation (LUNA) or presacral neurectomy (PSN) depending on which nerves are targeted.*[106]

104 "How is Endometriosis Treated?" Endometriosis.net; Sun-Wei Guo, "Recurrence of endometriosis and its control," *Human Reproduction Update* 15, no. 4 (March 2009): 441; "Endometriosis: Recurrence and Surgical Management," Cleveland Clinic, last modified August 1, 2014.

105 "How do healthcare providers diagnose endometriosis?" National Institute of Health, last modified February 21, 2020.

106 "How is Endometriosis Treated?" Endometriosis.net; "Uterine Nerve Ablation (UNA) and Presacral Neurectomy (PSN)," Aetna, last modified December 4, 2019.

Again, even more invasive surgeries do not guarantee the complete eradication of endometriosis symptoms.[107]

In addition to more traditional avenues, women with endometriosis will also often try alternative treatments, such as:

- acupuncture
- chiropractic care
- herbal medicine
- and mind-body practices like yoga and meditation.[108]

As there is no cure, these complementary therapies can help sufferers manage their symptoms and pain outside of their standard medical care and provide relief on a more day-to-day basis.[109]

***

In the case of vaginismus, as the underlying cause can be both a physical and mental issue, treatment can involve both sex therapy and physical therapy.

---

107 "How is Endometriosis Treated?" Endometriosis.net; "Hysterectomy," The American College of Obstetricians and Gynecologists, accessed June 20, 2020.

108 "How is Endometriosis Treated?" Endometriosis.net.

109 Ibid.

Sex therapy is often centered around unpacking underlying psychological issues or irrational and incorrect beliefs about sex.[110]

Physical therapy treatments often consist of dilation techniques involving a set of vaginal trainers which increase in size and length that a patient can use on their own time to gradually train the vaginal muscles to relax. Other physical exercises involving breathing exercises and progressive relaxation where you practice relaxing different muscles of the body one at a time, including tensing and relaxing your pelvic floor muscles.[111]

Fear of penetration is often not solely relegated to sexual encounters for many vaginismus sufferers, though. As in both Savannah and Lara's cases, the condition may cause gynecological examinations to be extremely painful, leading to a phobia of medical or clinical vaginal exams.[112]

Internal vaginal examinations are common in women's and AFAB individual's health plans, used for contraceptives (IUD), for ultrasounds (to check for health complications in the uterus/ovaries or for pregnancy-related exams), to accompany medical investigations, for smear tests (cervical screening test to help prevent cancer), and so on.[113] Some sufferers may find their muscles more relaxed in a medical setting, and may find these

---

110 "Vaginismus," Health Service Executive.

111 Ibid.

112 "The Vaginismus Network's Guide," Vaginismus Network.

113 "Smear Tests," Vaginismus Network, accessed October 2, 2020; "What is cervical screening?" National Health Service accessed October 2, 2020.

examinations bearable. But for those who find medical exams impossible or massively painful, regular health checkups can become traumatic and health warning signs may be missed.

Smear tests, for example, are generally recommended to be performed every three years beginning around the age of twenty-one and require the insertion of a speculum to collect cells from the cervix[114]. Some sufferers choose to deal with their "fear of the smear" by just ignoring the test, especially if they are considered low risk for cervical cancer.[115] But there are better ways for the medical community to handle exam phobia.

The Vaginismus Network has outlined a guide to help sufferers feel more in control of the process and help medical professionals find new avenues with which they can proceed with the exam. Some key points include:

Appointment preparation:

- set up a separate appointment to first discuss the procedure
- offer a speculum for the patient to practice with at home
- ask the patient if they would like to bring someone as support to the appointment

Relaxation/distraction:

- mindful breathing: long breaths in and out of the stomach
- listening to music, a podcast, a TV show, etc. may help

---

114 "Pap smear," Mayo Clinic, accessed October 2, 2020.
115 "Smear Tests," Vaginismus Network.

- over-the-counter relaxation remedies or prescribed medical relaxation aids

Upon arrival:

- ask the patient if they want to insert the speculum themselves
- preferably use the smallest size speculum possible
- ask the patient if they would prefer to lie on their side with their knees curled up (fetal position)
- if the patient is on their back, putting a pillow under the hips can help the pelvis open
- use lubrication

During the test

- does the patient want to be talked through what's happening during the exam?
- would the patient prefer it to be fast, slow, or particularly gentle?

After the test

- if the patient is distressed, offer them somewhere to sit quietly with water
- provide helpful resources (i.e. sex therapist, physical therapist, etc.)
- if the test is unsuccessful, discuss what they may want to try next time
- if the test is too traumatic for the patient, general anesthetic can be considered/discussed[116]

---

116 "The Vaginismus Network's Guide," Vaginismus Network.

Recognizing the legitimate psychosexual condition vaginismus sufferers are dealing with (i.e. not chalking it up to nerves, telling the patient to "just relax," or ignoring signs of fear) and understanding each vaginismus patient is different with different needs can result in a more positive and successful exam experience.[117]

The power of information and destigmatization regarding vaginal pain issues cannot be understated. Diagnosis and treatment are achieved by arming people with the necessary education to recognize their symptoms of an underlying condition and by properly and explicitly training medical professionals on vaginal pain conditions. Moreover, creating an environment in which women and AFAB individuals feel comfortable expressing their concerns to a provider, a parent, a partner, etc., promotes a healthy view of vaginal health as important to overall health.

We're beginning to see the power of education and demystification of these conditions: endometriosis is gradually gaining traction as a more widely known term. We're even starting to see ads specifically geared toward this issue which encourage sufferers to talk with their doctors if they're experiencing said symptoms. Vaginismus, though less known among the general public, reports a 95 percent treatment success rate in most clinical trials due to the variety of therapy solutions available.[118]

---

117 Ibid.
118 Michelle Kukla, "Vaginismus: What It Is and How It Can Be Treated," Good Therapy, March 27, 2018; Vaginismus Awareness, accessed October 2, 2020.

Yet, another so-called "V-problem"—vulvodynia—is far less researched, its causes are inconclusive or unknown, and its treatment nowhere near 100 percent effective. Equally as physically and emotionally damaging as endometriosis and vaginismus can be, why does vulvodynia remain such a mystery?

CHAPTER 5

The Intimacy Tax

Scrunching her toes, Fiona rolled over onto her side, tucking her elbow underneath her pillow. She watched his back rise and fall with each inhale and exhale as the sun peeked through the blinds. In their haste, they had forgotten to close them last night. Thinking of last night brought a smile to her lips.

The ceremony had been lovely. They invited just a few close family members and friends to attend the wedding and everything had gone smoothly. At eighteen, they couldn't shell out for a fancy party, but Fiona had looked glorious in her dress, the DIY decorations sparkled, and the home-cooked meal was worthy of three Michelin stars. They had stayed up late drinking and dancing and laughing until everyone's feet were sore, throats were hoarse, and speech a little slurred. The night ebbing, her husband finally carried her off, the sound of raucous hooting following them to bed.

It was here Fiona's smile dropped. Their first night as husband and wife was supposed to be special—certain "expectations" to be upheld. It had also been Fiona's first time, and though she had been expecting it to be uncomfortable, even a little painful (it always was the first time, wasn't it?), she hadn't expected it to hurt so much.

She also hadn't expected it to feel like she was being singed from the inside out.

Needless to say, it was a disappointing end to the night for them both. Shaking away the memory, Fiona decided not to dwell on it anymore. After all, the first time hurt for every woman, so said everyone. Next time would be much better.

***

Weeks went by, and the pain remained. It seemed even the slightest touch brought a fire roaring to life between her legs. Even wearing the wrong pair of pants or sitting in a car with the seat angled just so could send the pain shooting up her spine. When she began jumping away every time her husband reached for her, Fiona decided it was time to go see a gynecologist.

The first doctor told her it was nothing to worry about, that it was common for women to be uncomfortable during sex because they might be holding on to internalized ideas about sex being "dirty" or "wrong."

The next doctor told her to take a hot bath and have a glass of wine to relax.

The next and the next and the next told her she was crazy, and it was all in her head.

Pretty soon, Fiona started to wonder if it really was all in her head. She had no reason to distrust her medical professionals' expertise. She was no doctor herself. So, began the self-doubt:

"What's the matter with me?"

"Am I crazy? Am I imagining it?"

"*Is* there some kind of unhealthy idea I have, in fact, internalized about sex or about my husband?"

But as soon as those ideas would run through her head, or as soon as she would take their advice and drink a glass of wine, the pain would shoot through her again, reminding her of its realness.

"So, you have these two competing ideas in your head," Fiona says, "and it kind of creates a lot of cognitive dissonance and it creates a doubt and a mistrust in your own self because now you're not even trusted to know if your own experiences are true."

The lack of treatment and validation began to take a toll on Fiona's mental health and her relationship with her body. She slowly started to disconnect from her body, and she stopped trusting her intuition. She didn't want to be touched; she was afraid to even touch herself. Her sense of intimacy with her husband deteriorated before it even had the chance to flourish, and though he was always supportive and never pressed her, the constant rejection of sexual advances left him feeling unwanted and undesired.

Without any diagnosis or hope for a fix, Fiona's situation worsened when the couple started trying to conceive. The repeated painful sexual experiences began to mess with Fiona's pelvic floor as each time, with the anticipation of pain, her muscles clenched and re-clenched. The nerves near her hymen had also been damaged from childhood abuse, and these damaged nerves were sending additional messages of "Danger! Danger!" to her brain. As a result, her pelvic floor muscles were stretched and shortened every which way, putting pressure on her ovaries and interfering with her menstruation.

This set off a string of other complications: first she got really sick, and then had difficulty conceiving, and then had several miscarriages. More and more, Fiona felt as if she didn't fit the definition of a whole, healthy, functioning woman because she was failing at the most basic biological conditions of womanhood.

***

Fiona and her husband divorced several years ago, but Fiona sees the idea of dating again as almost impossible.

"What kind of potential partner is going to want to date a woman who possibly cannot have an intimate relationship or have children or create a family together, which is generally what people want when they get married?" she wonders.

She says it feels as if she might not be able to have the future she envisioned, or as if her future might be on hold.

For a while it seemed as if that might be the case. After doctor after doctor dismissed her throughout her twenties, after trying hormone-balancing diets and testosterone-suppressing medication, after hearing, "*Yes*, there is something wrong with you, but *no* you're imagining pain during sex" a million and one times, after having to rely on her husband attending her appointments to be taken seriously in the slightest, she finally stopped.

She stopped all the medications which weren't helping and were sometimes hurting.

She stopped seeking out more doctors who were just going to tell her she was crazy again.

Even as she thought, *I'm going to have to live with this forever*, Fiona noticed her mental health improving. On a whim, she decided to join a Facebook support group for women's pelvic pain. In that group there was a woman who shared her story, including how she got a diagnosis for her condition. Her symptoms and condition were different from Fiona's, but *this woman* had a *diagnosis—**a diagnosis acknowledging she had pain in her pelvic region.***

So, Fiona reached out to this female enigma and asked her *How?*

How did you get a diagnosis?

How did you get a doctor to listen to you and trust you and offer you a diagnosis?

How did that happen?

The woman emailed Fiona back and said she had had similar experiences with doctors and recommended a book on physical therapy that might help. That book, though it steered her in the right direction, sent Fiona on another long journey where she finally received a diagnosis of vulvodynia a year-and-a-half ago at the age of thirty-four after having symptoms her entire life.

> *Vulvodynia is a very general term used for chronic, unexplained vulvar pain. The pain differs in constancy, location, and severity among sufferers.*[119]

The most commonly described symptoms are:

- Burning
- Stinging
- Irritation
- Soreness
- Aching
- Swelling[120]

For some it feels like a blister rubbing raw on the skin, for others it can feel like "acid being poured on the skin" or "constant knife-like pain."[121]

Vulvodynia can also be categorized into two subtypes: **localized** and **generalized:**

---

119 "What is Vulvodynia?" National Vulvodynia Association accessed June 14, 2020.

120 "Vulvodynia," The American College of Obstetricians and Gynecologists, accessed June 14, 2020.

121 "What is Vulvodynia?" National Vulvodynia Association.

*With **localized** vulvodynia, the sufferer experiences pain in one specific area. For example, experiencing pain in the tissue surrounding the vaginal opening is described as vestibulodynia, and pain in the clitoris is known as clitorodynia.[122] For most women with localized symptoms, pain arises during or after pressure is applied to the area, which can range from penetration to wearing fitted pants.[123]*

*With **generalized** vulvodynia, pain occurs more spontaneously and is not always specific to one area, potentially spreading as far as the top of legs or inner thighs. Though the pain is more constant with some periods of relief, certain activities which apply pressure to the area typically worsen symptoms.[124]*

Though the cause of vulvodynia is not known, and does differ between sufferers, researchers believe some underlying causes may be:

- Injury or irritation of nerves that transmit pain signals from the vulva to the spinal cord
- An increase in numbers or sensitivity of pain-sensing nerve fibers in the vulva
- An increase in inflammatory substances in the vulva

---

122 "What is Vulvodynia?" National Vulvodynia Association; "Vulvodynia," The American College of Obstetricians and Gynecologists.

123 "What is Vulvodynia?" National Vulvodynia Association.

124 "What is Vulvodynia?" National Vulvodynia Association; Sy Kraft, "Vulvodynia: What you need to know," Medical News Today, March 13, 2017.

- An abnormal response from vulvar cells to infection or trauma
- Genetic susceptibility
- Pelvic floor muscle dysfunction.[125]

The exact prevalence of vulvar pain is not known, but studies suggest 16 percent of women in the US suffer from vulvodynia during their lifetime.[126] According to a study funded by the National Institutes of Health, nearly 60 percent of sufferers cannot have sexual intercourse due to pain or anticipation of pain, and 75 percent feel "out of control" of their bodies.[127] As a result, vulvodynia can take a serious toll on a sufferer's mental health and self-image, just as it had for so long with Fiona.

Fiona did so much research in the ten-plus years she was looking for answers, she says she feels like a doctor herself. She also found so many additional stories of women who similarly had been repeatedly invalidated by their health care providers, who had been diagnosed with an emotional issue, who had to bring their partners in to appointments to testify as witness to their pain.

---

125 "What is Vulvodynia?" National Vulvodynia Association; "Vulvodynia," The American College of Obstetricians and Gynecologists.

126 Kraft, "Vulvodynia"; Bernard L. Harlow and Elizabeth Gunther Stewart, "A population-based assessment of chronic unexplained vulvar pain: have we underestimated the prevalence of vulvodynia?" *Journal of the American Medical Women›s Association* 58, no. 2 (January 2003): 82.

127 Lauren D. Arnold et al., "Assessment of Vulvodynia Symptoms in a Sample of U.S. Women: A Prevalence Survey with a Nested Case Control Study," *American Journal of Obstetrics and Gynecology* 196, no. 2 (February 2007): 3.

"It was very infantilizing to [feel like] I cannot be trusted as an adult to report on my own experiences and I need someone else there to validate me," she says, "but it was shocking, and also somewhat comforting, to know I'm not the only one. Because otherwise you feel so alone."

For years, Fiona's doctors told her the pain she felt during sex was not normal and she was alone in her experience, when in reality there are millions of women in the US alone who deal with these issues every day. In fact, it is estimated dyspareunia, which causes recurrent or persistent pain with sexual activity, affects 10-20 percent of US women.[128] *Fiona thinks one of the biggest things which would make her pain feel more manageable would be being able to openly and shamelessly talk about it.*

Over the past two years, Fiona has had three hip surgeries most likely necessitated because of her pelvic floor dysfunction. The surgeries put her in a huge brace and she had to use crutches, and she noticed people felt very comfortable coming up to her and asking her, "Oh did you break your leg, did you hurt you hip?" and then would tell her about the time they broke their foot skiing or fractured their leg playing soccer.

"They feel very comfortable talking about these traumatic physical experiences because they are in non-taboo parts of the human body," Fiona observes, "but talking about your vulva or your vaginal pain is very taboo, and not

---

128 Dean A. Seehusen, Drew C. Baird, and David V. Bode, "Dyspareunia in Women," *American Family Physician* 90, no. 7 (October 2014): 465.

just taboo, but also very intimate. It's connected to our most intimate part of what it means to be a woman or how we can experience our womanhood. So, sometimes I think not being able to talk about it is what causes a lot of my emotional pain, which actually feels worse than the physical pain itself and certainly exacerbates it, as I feel so alone in this."

It's this lack of communication and awareness around issues considered too "uncomfortable" which leaves people dealing with vaginal or vulvar pain feeling so alone. For Fiona, finding a diagnosis helped to dispel some of those feelings because she found the validation from medical providers and fellow sufferers she had been actively seeking for years. *It felt like her pain was finally being recognized.*

Failing to recognize or believe pain in female sexual health, whether it be in the medical field or general education, is damaging to an individual's physical health, mental health, and sense of sexuality. Underlying the dismissal and invalidation is the normalization of female pain—the idea sex and periods and reproduction hurts every uterus and vagina, so it must hurt every person the same.

If it hurts every person the same, no female has the right or grounds for complaint.

What we end up with then, are girls, women, and AFAB individuals who experience intense pain and think it's normal, who think pain is biologically written into their DNA as a carrier of a vagina, and therefore is their cross to bear.

On the one hand, we have women like Fiona, who desperately search for answers to something they know is wrong; on the other hand, we have women like Vera, who realize something is wrong only *after* someone finally says, "Wait, sex feels like *what* to you?"

***

TW: Rape.

When Vera was twelve and tried inserting a tampon for the first time and felt an excruciating burning between her legs, she thought it was normal.

When Vera was fourteen and had sex for the first time and it felt like she was being ripped apart again and again, she thought that's what every girl or woman felt their first time.

When Vera had to ask her boyfriend to stop right in the middle because the pain was more than she could handle, and then he dumped her a few days later, she blamed herself for insisting he stop and fell into a suicidal depression.

Vera resolved from then on to undergo the sexual process all the way, no matter what. She didn't want her lack of execution to ruin any future relationships. She figured she just needed to push through, that this was just part of being a woman.

It wasn't until her early twenties an older friend finally clued Vera in, telling her the level of pain she was experiencing was not normal. The discovery she might have an underlying condition, that not every woman or person with a vagina experienced intense pain or deep discomfort with sex, tampons, or speculum exams, was a double-edged sword for Vera.

On the one hand, she had managed to bear the burden for years—to be what she thought it meant to be a "full" woman and live what she thought was a normal sex life. On the other hand, she had been repeatedly forcing herself to experience less-than-pleasant sexual encounters *because* no one had ever informed her the pain wasn't normal.

Upon gynecological examination, the physical appearance of her pelvic and vaginal region presented healthy. Without follow-up probing questions about pain or other sensations in the area to uncover potential issues, Vera and her doctors remained unaware she suffered from vulvodynia. At best, when doctors noticed her tensing during exams, she was told to relax, but no one asked her if she was feeling any pain, either during the exam or during sexual activity.

Vera's case is interesting because her vulvodynia did not prevent her from having sexual intercourse. She physically would push through the pain, which is likely due to the level of severity of her condition compared to others, and because sex was nevertheless a way for Vera to experience a profound type of intimacy.

She says, "Even before I knew there was a problem, sex was the epitome of closeness for me. Due to the pain, sex could never just be light and casual. It required an extreme level of trust and a codependent level of closeness. I was entrusting my partner with my deepest suffering and that was profoundly intimate. This was not a romantic notion; rather it was a psychological necessity that made painful sex possible."

To let someone in on her pain was the extent of Vera's understanding of what a normal, pleasurable sexual experience should feel like.

Later in life, though, she has taken a step back to evaluate her relationship with her sexuality.

Living in a culture which seems to place an emphasis on sex at every turn, sexual dysfunction can start to feel like your central identity. For Vera, she says because of her challenging sex life, her "self-worth was wrapped up in sex," and dealing with these issues can "swallow you up." In a hyper-sexualized society, your worth is threatened by an inability to lead a "normal" sex life.

When every sexual encounter you have is laced with pain, when every experience requires effort and attention and is mentally and physically impactful, when you can never have sex in a relaxed, casual way, your sense of sexuality can feel throttled.

This is how her condition truly impacted Vera. The physical pain she could barrel through if she needed to, but the potential emotional pain of being rejected for her inability to sexually perform was devastating. From her experiences and childhood impression of society, Vera lived believing to be accepted and fully loved as a romantic partner she had to endure the sexual pain which made it possible. While she eventually healed that belief, there is now a weight to her sexual identity. A burden she has to carry and share with romantic partners.

"While I now have a sense of self no longer rooted and dependent on my sexual performance, sex can never just be easy and carefree."

There is a boundary, to some extent, on her physical pain that doesn't exist with emotional pain. Even if you have people in your life who want to share that emotional load with you, it can still feel extremely isolating because they could never truly understand.

"I feel like each person is an island," Vera says about sufferers, "an island with their own internal version of the external story."

Particularly, with such a sensitive, taboo topic, opening up about it can be additionally difficult, further cementing a sufferer's sense of isolation. It can feel shameful and humiliating to even bring it up with your doctor because sexual issues are kept so "hush-hush" throughout adolescence and into adulthood, and because of a pervasive belief society expects a healthy "normal."

But any young woman thinking painful sex or pain with using period products is the singular experience is unacceptable. There are measures of pain, and there are differences between pain and discomfort.

Why are women and AFAB individuals not being taught how to recognize pain related to sexual health issues with our bodies? This pain, left untreated and unacknowledged, can bleed into our functionality on a daily basis, our romantic relationships, and our emotional health.

Vera is a prime example of how our current narrative on female pain lends itself to the idea women just need to push through it—to just deal with it, even if you are pushing yourself to have sexual experiences you don't want, or do want but will not enjoy.

"If you're accepting pain with sex, that's not very different than being raped," Vera argues. "The worst part about it, though, is that you, yourself, are having to consent to your own rape in order to feel normal in society, or 'okay' as a human being. I think that's the most fucked up thing about it. You literally have to be your own rapist."

Why should that ever be deemed acceptable? Vaginal and vulvar pain issues are broader than getting validation or a diagnosis from a doctor or understanding they exist.

The female pain narrative needs to be reformatted. Depending on the severity or nature of each individual's condition, different accommodations for sex or sexual health exams work for different people.

But why are we telling women sex *should* hurt?

Why are we perpetuating this belief the pleasure or needs of their partner is more important than their physical and mental comfort and safety?

Sex does not only occur between a penis and vagina. It is not an activity which needs to, or always does, involve penetration. It also should *never* involve any sort of activity that makes any person uncomfortable. By placing pressure on women to engage in penetrative sexual activities, especially those in heterosexual relationships or relationships involving a penis and vagina, it reinforces the idea that the only "real" sex is penis-in-vagina sex. This delegitimizes the sexual experiences of the LGBTQ+ community and signals to women dealing with vaginal pain issues that an integral part of their womanhood is "broken."

Sex ed should not just focus on how sex works and what the consequences may be. It should also focus on the parameters within which sex should function. Explain consent, explain pleasure, explain if you are in pain it is absolutely okay to stop. Reframing sex ed conversations around what healthy sexual health experiences actually look like, whether that be with periods, sex, gynecology exams, etc., establishes an awareness of one's self to know when something is off and needs attention in a way which destigmatizes the issue.

CHAPTER 6

It's Not PMS

Monday dawned and Courtney blearily opened her eyes to the sound of her alarm clock. She glared at the sunlight filtering through her shades, seeming far too cheerful for her mood this morning. Grumbling, it took all her effort to drag herself out of bed and start her pre-work routine.

But nothing seemed to want to go her way that morning. Her hair wouldn't lie flat, her coffee lid wouldn't screw on correctly, and there were dishes in the sink. She felt her anger fizzling with each inconvenience.

As she drove to work and someone in front of her moved too slowly through a green light, Courtney felt it spark.

As she arrived at work and someone didn't hold the elevator for her, she felt it boil over.

God is the world just against me today? she seethed.

Courtney could feel herself being irrational, which only served to provoke her frustration as she failed again and again to maintain control over her spiking emotions. Finally, she snapped.

Courtney arrived just a few minutes late to the meeting, hurriedly taking her seat to join the conference call. This was a big meeting for her department, and it was important for her to remain in the right headspace. Taking a calming breath, she turned her attention to her boss, who was giving Courtney a proper introduction.

Dipping her head in response, Courtney launched into her prepared speech on the new development project for Staten Island. Not a minute in, and the speaker in the middle of the table crackled with the promise of an interjection from someone on the other end of the call.

"Uh, ya, I think you meant to say $1,500 instead of $3,500. No way it would cost that much," came a man's voice over the phone.

Shaking her head, Courtney double-checked her spreadsheet. "No, I've got the estimates right here," she replied. "We've worked with these guys in the past, and for two months it would be $3,500. But we can discuss more after I go through the rest of the numbers."

She continued, grimacing when she heard the tell-tale crackling as he stepped in to interrupt again, and again, and again.

"No, no, that's not right."

"Ya, you didn't mean to say that."

"Well, based on *my* calculations..."

Courtney felt a jab of rage shoot up her spine every time this man spoke. Granted, he was being a jerk, but she needed to remain professional and keep her thoughts to herself. Swallowing her distaste, she responded to each interruption through gritted teeth.

"I understand why you may think that," she said, "but if you just let me explain how my team and I got these..."

"I just don't see these numbers adding up," he stopped her again. "Let's take a look at the timeline we've developed because that's a better indicator..."

This time it was Courtney interrupting, her reaction sudden as her blood boiled over.

"No, please, you speak," she patronized. "You're the man, I'm just a woman. I'll just sit here and be quiet."

As Courtney spit out the insult, the rush of sudden silence slapped her back to reality. She blinked away the spots of fury to find a dozen shocked faces staring back at her. Hot-faced, she quickly excused herself, wondering how she had just managed to lose her self-control like that.

Though this was a dramatic example, one which didn't cost Courtney her job but did land her an HR violation, it certainly wasn't the first time she had involuntarily lashed out, felt depressive, or irrationally irritable.

Courtney suffers from a condition called premenstrual dysphoric disorder (PMDD).

> *According to the International Association for Pre-menstrual Disorders (IAPMD), PMDD is "a cyclical, hormone-based mood disorder with symptoms arising during the premenstrual, or luteal phase of the menstrual cycle and lasting until the onset of menstrual flow."*[129]

While PMDD is a disorder linked to the period cycle, it is a suspected cellular disorder in the brain, not a hormone imbalance. In a 2017 study, researchers at the National Institutes of Health found women and AFAB individuals with PMDD experience severe negative reactions to natural changes in estrogen and progesterone during the luteal phase, which may be due to their genetic molecular processing systems.[130]

> *The luteal phase is the second half of the menstrual cycle when the body prepares for pregnancy. The phase begins after ovulation and ends with the first day of menstruation, which lasts 12 to 14 days for most women.*[131]

---

129 "What is PMDD?" International Association for Premenstrual Disorders, last modified January 14, 2019.

130 "What is PMDD?" International Association for Premenstrual Disorders; National Institutes of Health, "Sex hormone-sensitive gene complex linked to premenstrual mood disorder," Medical Xpress, January 3, 2017.

131 "All About the Luteal Phase of the Menstrual Cycle," Healthline, accessed September 8, 2020; Tolga B. Mesen and Steven L. Young, "Progesterone and the Luteal Phase: A Requisite to Reproduction," *Obstetrics and Gynecology Clinics of North America* 42, no. 1 (March 2015): 138.

Simply put, PMDD is believed to be an "abnormal response to normal hormonal changes."[132]

The condition is predicted to affect anywhere from 5–10 percent of women and AFAB individuals of reproductive age—approximately three to six million women/AFAB in the US—and is characterized by a slew of emotional and physical symptoms.[133] Some of the most prevalent include:

- depression
- anxiety
- suicidal thoughts
- extreme mood swings
- frequent crying
- lasting irritability and anger
- fatigue
- trouble sleeping
- headaches
- amnesia
- and bloating.[134]

Symptoms can appear at a young age, but often worsen overtime and especially around reproductive events, such as pregnancy, birth, miscarriage, and perimenopause.[135]

---

132 Edwin R. Raffi and Marlene P. Freeman, "The etiology of premenstrual dysphoric disorder: 5 interwoven pieces," *Current Psychiatry* 16, no. 9 (September 2017): 26; Peter J. Schmidt et al., "Differential behavioral effects of gonadal steroids in women with and in those without premenstrual syndrome," *New England Journal of Medicine* 338, no. 4 (January 22, 1998): 209.

133 "About PMDD," International Association for Premenstrual Disorders, last modified March 21, 2019.

134 "What is PMDD?" International Association for Premenstrual Disorders.

135 Ibid.

Though PMDD is often confused with, or diagnosed as, premenstrual syndrome (PMS), the two differ. PMS also comprises a mix of emotional and physical symptoms, including bloating, weepiness, and irritability, and is often used as a dismissive explanation in popular culture for a woman's "moodiness" or volatile behavior.

However, while PMS can also disrupt a woman's quality of life, impact her ability to attend work or school, and impede her relationships, PMS is more easily managed and presents less severe symptoms than PMDD. Additionally, PMS is not classified as a mental illness, whereas PMDD is listed in the Diagnostic and Statistical Manual of Mental Disorders, 5th Edition (DSM-5).[136]

The similarities to PMS make PMDD difficult to diagnose and the underlying molecular and chemical nature of the condition make it even more difficult to treat; the severity of symptoms and life-threatening consequences necessitate more education and awareness surrounding this issue.

Many sufferers describe living with PMDD like living a "half-life," or say it can feel like "one week of hell and three weeks of cleaning up" due to damaging and impulsive behaviors, such as suddenly leaving a job or relationship.[137] Not only is the condition emotionally and professionally destructive, but physically threatening when thoughts of suicide and self-harm arise.

---

136 Ibid.
137 Ibid.

An estimated 15–30 percent of women and AFAB individuals with PMDD attempt suicide, with an even larger percentage having suicidal and self-harm thoughts.[138]

Courtney is one such sufferer who routinely has had suicidal thoughts during a cycle of PMDD, and who has seen the damage her condition can cause with personal and professional relationships. But for decades, she had no answer as to why she seemed to turn into a different person sometimes. For years it was confused as other things or treated incorrectly.

She was prescribed birth control, which doctors said would help her hormones stabilize, but resulted in her symptoms becoming more sporadic throughout the month rather than being concentrated for the week or two before her period.

She was prescribed antidepressants, but later found those were not improving her symptoms at all.

Four years ago, after her pregnancy, Courtney's symptoms worsened as she dealt with postpartum depression on top of her PMDD. "I was going through just a terrible time emotionally and I could not understand why," she recalls.

She eventually chanced upon several PMDD support groups with stories from women exhibiting similar symptoms and sharing similar experiences to Courtney's. As she dug further, and began to track the timing of her symptoms, she slowly

---

138 "About PMDD," International Association for Premenstrual Disorders; "Treating premenstrual dysphoric disorder," Harvard Health Publishing, last modified July 30, 2019.

started to understand her condition. It was thanks to these women and Courtney's own intuition she was finally able to uncover the name and cause for her symptoms.

Courtney is fortunate: she discovered her condition and was able to seek specialist help for it. She did not become a statistic. She is especially lucky because her PMDD has improved leaps and bounds since introducing her treatment and medication.

She began going to a local psychiatry practice every month in New York City which focuses on women's reproductive mental health. Every session they talk about how the last month went, go over the game plan for the coming cycle, and remind Courtney what her prescription is doing for her and why it's important for her to take it regularly. The sessions are helpful to prepare Courtney for her next cycle and to ensure she feels in control. She may not be able to control a lot of her emotions when she's in the middle of PMDD, but she can make an active choice to take her medication every day, which helps her sleep and reduces the severity of her symptoms.

A large part of her motivation to find and stick with a treatment comes from her son. "I never want to lash out at him and I'm not a yeller with him," Courtney says, "but there's been a couple of times when I've snapped at him and his little lip quivers and he'll ask me, 'What, why did you yell? I was listening.' And it just breaks my heart."

He serves as a constant reminder for her to take her medication, even when she feels like maybe it's not necessary that day.

"I was always fighting the idea I needed to take medication. So even though my doctor would say, 'Okay this is your regimen,' I would still be like, 'let's just see though if I really need it.'"

But every time Courtney would lash out and make her kid cry, she would feel guilty afterwards. Now, she's made a pact with herself to take her prescription every day, and though it's not a 100 percent fix, she's never felt better.

One of the greatest comforts for Courtney, which is echoed again and again, is the support she finds from groups of women sharing their stories online.

"It's life changing just to know there are so many other women who are going through this and who are just discovering it for the first time," says Courtney, " and to be in a position to share my experience and help somebody, but also to be helped by somebody. I think the biggest thing is feeling like this is a legitimate thing, and not something that you're making up."

Gia Allemand, an American actress who died in 2013, was a good friend of one of Courtney's childhood friends. Gia was a sufferer of PMDD and took her own life, it is believed, during one of her bouts. Courtney, reflecting on the tragedy, expresses, "I guess it really hit home to me that this woman arguably committed suicide during a temporary state of insanity, which I feel like I go through every month."

Prior to her diagnosis, Courtney had no idea that a cellular disorder was the cause of her temporarily altered state of mind, and without receiving that diagnosis she very well may have sought a similar escape. Sometimes all she needs is a little reassurance she's not crazy, and her negative feelings will pass, to get her through.

"If I didn't know it was PMDD and I didn't know it was cyclical and temporary, I might be Gia Allemand," she cautions. A grim statement, but an all-too-real reason why education and awareness surrounding PMDD is so incredibly vital. Generalizing the symptoms of all menstrual cycles to fit into an easy lesson for sex ed class, which we carry with us into adulthood, creates a very singular definition of how different people experience their cycle.

***

We are taught that periods suck. Sure it's great the first time because it means "Ta-da, you're a woman!," but then they're a pain, and uncomfortable, and a burden women just have to bear.

When we hear things like, "She's just PMSing," and, "Ooh, looks like it's that time of the month again, huh?"—remarks meant to minimize and invalidate women's emotions—it normalizes, diminishes, and makes a joke of very real, involuntary hormone fluctuations. Beyond the obviously problematic issue of likening all emotional female behavior to their periods, messages of this sort make it easy to write off symptoms of PMDD as nothing more than the regular monthly trials of womanhood. Medical professionals, too, will stick to the mantra that it's just PMS, every woman goes through this, and that if you're complaining, you're just milking it.

When PMDD begins at a younger age, or is all you've known since your first period, it can be especially difficult to distinguish your symptoms from the PMS symptoms 90 percent of people who have periods experience. Expressing concerns over something everyone else thinks is raging teen hormones creates an additional barrier to the recognition of a deeper issue.

Such was the case for Caroline, whose symptoms started in seventh grade, about two years after she got her period for the first time. She didn't really start to pick up on them until a couple of months later, however, as she began sleeping less and less, growing more fatigued and more irritable.

She checks a lot of the boxes for PMDD symptoms, both physically and emotionally. Every month for the past three to four years she has suffered from bouts of headaches, fatigue, bloating, insomnia, sensitivity to light, inability to concentrate, amnesia, heightened sensitivity to rejection, irritability, depression, anxiety, and suicidal thoughts.

When she first began to notice something was off toward the end of middle school, she wasn't sure what was wrong, if there even was anything wrong, or what to do about it. She was riding a wild rollercoaster of emotions already fraught with the accompanying twists and turns of puberty and middle school upheavals.

Caroline describes her PMDD like, "being smacked in the face with a pan once a month, or like having ADHD, or going on a Xanax withdrawal for a week before your period."

She tried to talk to her friends about it, but without knowing what was wrong and without the vocabulary to express herself, she could only describe it as feeling absolutely miserable one day and then fantastic the next.

"Ya, that's puberty for you," was all she got in response.

Even once she eventually tied her emotional discrepancies to the timing of her periods:

"Okay, but I have really, really bad periods too," she tried again.

"Everyone gets bad periods, but I guess we just deal with it better than you do. Stop being so dramatic."

Even her primary care doctors shoved off her concerns when she brought up her symptoms and rocky emotions. Much to her frustration, they continually chalked it up to just a normal part of being a teenager and told her she needed to figure out a way to handle those intense highs and lows.

It wasn't until months after her symptoms first appeared she realized something really was wrong—it couldn't possibly be normal puberty stuff.

Her last year of middle school, she and her classmates had the exciting opportunity to participate in a foreign exchange program in Mexico City for a week.

Unfortunately, that week coincided with one of the worst weeks in her cycle.

She was staying with a very nice host family, learning a lot, exploring a fascinating city, but everything felt off. Every little thing set her on edge, and she felt constantly flushed with anger. She recalls becoming unreasonably enraged over mundane, everyday annoyances that set off a series of irrational thought processes and quickly spiraled into frustration and anger.

Her temper flared with little provocation, her exasperation often turning to barely-held-back tears. Embarrassed, and a little homesick, her mind wreaking havoc on her emotions, she got into a lot of fights over the course of that week.

"It felt like all hell broke loose," she says, "and it kind of just drove me crazy."

Help for her condition remained elusive, though. Recognizing her symptoms had something to do with her period felt like a step in the right direction for her. Holding on to that one crucial discovery, she plodded through another shaky year, dreading every period but at least knowing they had something to do with her violent mood swings.

One night, nearing the end of her first year of high school, she finally decided enough was enough—she couldn't live like this anymore, pretending everything was normal. Snatching her laptop from her bed, she sat down at her desk and got to work. Not knowing what she was looking for, she started typing her symptoms into the search bar.

Period anger.

Depression and periods.

Painful periods.

Mood swings before my period.

The words premenstrual syndrome flashed across the screen, but she ignored them, knowing it was more than PMS, and dug deeper. Finally, she stumbled across the words which would answer her long-sought questions:

premenstrual dysphoric disorder

Her eyes roved impatiently over the symptoms, desperately needing them to be a match. *Severe irritability. Crying spells. Depression. Fatigue.* The list went on.

"I was refusing to believe I was just 'not handling things right.' I found PMDD and I checked every box on the list. I was just crying from relief; it was such an emotional moment for me."

It was late when she eventually surfaced from her hours of research. Padding downstairs, she found her mom in the kitchen.

"Mom?" she started, hesitated, trying to figure out how to form into words her newfound revelation.

"Mom, remember how I told you I get really emotional sometimes and I thought it had something to do with my period? I think there might be something more to it. I think I have something called PMDD. Can we book an appointment with the gynecologist?"

Fortunate enough to live close to New York City, there was no shortage of stellar doctors from top medical programs from which to choose. Her mom made the appointment, and shortly afterwards Caroline found herself in the gynecologist's office for the first time.

She had done her research and she was sure she needed help but faced with the uncertainty with which her adolescence had so far been plagued, her confidence faltered. She slipped back into the role she had played in front of doctors many times before.

"I don't think my emotions are normal," she told the doctor, half-expecting the same skepticism and blanket response she had heard every other time.

But instead, her doctor probed further, "Okay, so why don't you tell me some of your symptoms."

Caroline listed the ones she could remember from her research which fit her monthly ailments. Her doctor noted those down and then asked, "And do you have any of these?" She listed off additional symptoms, some of which Caroline remembers also reading and some she hadn't even realized were typical of the disorder.

"She knew what she was doing," Caroline comments about her gynecologist. "I was diagnosed within five minutes when I went to the right doctor."

Finally receiving affirmation and a concrete diagnosis was hugely relieving, but not an absolute cure. She was offered a couple of different treatment options and put on some medication, but since then her symptoms have only marginally improved.

PMDD is difficult to treat because it's molecular based and affects the chemicals in your brain. There is no umbrella treatment that works for everyone, or even for the majority of sufferers. Treatments have to be specified to the individual and their specific symptoms, and there is never a guarantee of immediate or eventual success.[139]

Yet, Caroline says it has been immensely beneficial, "just having the validation of knowing what I'm going through and knowing if I'm having a bad day my emotions are valid. Now I know I don't have to just stuff it down and pretend nothing's wrong, because that's what I used to think other girls were doing and they were just better at hiding it than me. So, I think my self-esteem has gone up a lot, even if the disorder itself hasn't gotten easier to deal with."

It's not a big ask to want our medical care givers and educators listen to women's concerns and properly educate them on their bodies, but it's so often simply not done. In the next chapter, we'll look deeper into why PMDD is decidedly easier to misdiagnose, and the severe consequences which can arise from ignoring the symptoms.

---

139 "Treatment Options," International Association for Premenstrual Disorders, last modified March 22, 2017.

CHAPTER 7

The Monster Within

PMDD is particularly difficult because it straddles sexual health and mental health, an area with which not a lot of medical professionals are familiar.

General practitioners may diagnose PMDD as a mental health issue and refer a patient to a psychologist, but then psychologists may view it as a physiological issue outside of their professional capabilities. They then point their patient back in the direction of a general practitioner or OB/GYN.

A lack of awareness and education can lead to a lot of battling back and forth between health care providers and often results in misdiagnosing PMDD as other mental health issues. As a result, health care professionals attempt to stitch together an explanation and fix based on erroneous or incomplete information and assumptions.

As we saw with Courtney and Caroline, ignoring or mischaracterizing PMDD is emotionally and physically damaging to sufferers.

> *According to the DSM-5, PMDD is defined as a depressive disorder, and as such can trigger lasting traumatic and life-threatening episodes.*[140]

As both a consistent and intermittent mental health disorder officially recognized as a mental disorder just seven years ago, PMDD is still widely misunderstood and under diagnosed.

This is expressly concerning when it presents its most vicious side.

***

"Hey babe, can you pass the salsa?"

Elena nodded distractedly and handed the bowl over to her partner Jordan, eyes glued to the TV. It was Sunday night and the game was on. Elena sneered as the quarterback was slammed into the ground from a surprise sack.

"Ha! You see that?" she exclaimed, stuffing a chip in her mouth.

"Ya, pass the chips too, please," Jordan replied.

"Oh, right, here you go."

"Ah shit," Jordan cursed as a glob of salsa dribbled onto their shirt. "You got a napkin or something over there I can use to..."

---

140 Raffi and Freeman, "The etiology of premenstrual," 21; American Psychiatric Association, *Diagnostic And Statistical Manual Of Mental Disorders, Fifth Edition* (Washington, DC: APA Press, 2013).

"Why do I have to do **everything** for you?" Elena burst out. "Can't I just watch the game? I just want to watch the game! It's like you don't even care! Do you even want to spend time with me?"

"What—no, I didn't mean..." Jordan tried before Elena cut him off again. She felt her face heating, her cheeks growing red as her irritation mounted. She was suddenly and inexorably angry—no, furious—at Jordan, at the game, at everything.

"Why are you being like this?" she screamed.

"I'm sorry, I don't understand what I did," Jordan placated.

"No, you *don't* understand, you don't *fucking* understand!"

On the verge of tears, she couldn't explain, Elena leapt from the couch and let out a stream of expletives as Jordan gaped up at her.

Frazzled, heart beating faster and faster as her adrenaline spiked, she spun around and tore through the house. She had to get away.

Elena felt her rage bubbling, felt it creep up her body and flow through her veins until she was shaking. It hit her brain and her fury sparked.

GAAAAAAAAGHHHHHH!

She screamed at the empty hallway. She knew she was screaming at someone, but suddenly she had forgotten who.

Spinning, she slammed the bedroom door shut, locking it behind her. Heaving, she desperately tried to cling to reason as her brain wrestled every logical thought out of her head, turning them to dust and fueling her rage until the connection snapped.

As if detached from her body, Elena watched herself turn and grab the nearest thing: a water bottle.

She watched as her wrist stiffened and her arm raise of its own volition.

She watched as her hand betrayed her, releasing the bottle mid-swing and sending it crashing full force into the door.

She watched as she bent down, scooped up the bottle, and prepared her next throw.

She watched herself hurl that bottle at the door again and again and again until the pounding noise beat like her own heartbeat and her vision went white.

When she came to, she was on the floor, the bruised bottle next to her. She flexed her treacherous hands. They were hers again.

Open, close, open, close.

Rotating her arm so her palm was facing up, she watched her tendons respond to her hand's movement. Taking a finger, she lightly traced a line across her wrist.

The vision was sudden and forceful.

A splice of red appeared where her finger had just been. Elena could see the cut and the blood just beginning to flow, and this time her body didn't let her go. She was trapped.

No, no, no, no, no.

Desperately, she swiped at her arm and tried to shake her head free of the vision, willing the torturous thoughts away.

A knock at the door tore her eyes away as her partner jiggled the locked door handle.

"Go!" Elena screamed. "Go away! Go away *now*! Leave me alone!"

I can't be seen like this—I can't. What's wrong with me?

Chest constricting and tears of anger and frustration threatening to spill, she glanced back at her wrist. The slit was gone.

***

Similar to flashbacks in post-traumatic stress disorder, Elena was experiencing mental imagery described as "flash-forwards" to suicide.

> *"Flash-forward" images are thought to be "involuntary, intrusive 'snapshots' of the suicidal acts...or the aftermath of suicide," which differs from voluntary thoughts or daydreaming about suicide.*[141]

However, though involuntary, several studies have linked mental imagery to an increased risk of, or more severe, suicidal ideation.[142] Just as other forms of mental imagery, like picturing yourself going to vote, can often act as a casual determinant for future behavior, there is growing evidence imagery as it relates to suicidal behavior may be similarly telling of future actions.[143]

At the very least, suicidal flash-forwards, as is the case for Elena, are often full of real and compelling sensory qualities comparable to the sensory-perceptual images of PTSD flashbacks, provoking episodes which feel very real and very traumatic.[144]

This area of research in suicidal behavior is still new and has not yet been studied specifically for PMDD sufferers. As a depressive disorder, however, it follows people like Elena who may experience the same level of intense suicidal imagery or ideation during their cycle as others undergoing depressive episodes.

---

141 Roger M.K. Ng et al., "'Flash-forwards' and suicidal ideation: A prospective investigation of mental imagery, entrapment and defeat in a cohort from the Hong Kong Mental Morbidity Survey," *Psychiatry Research* 246, no. 30 (December 2016): 454; Emily A. Holmes, "Imagery about suicide in depression—"Flash-forwards"?" *Journal of Behavior Therapy and Experimental Psychiatry* 38, no. 4 (December 2007): 423.

142 Ng et al., "'Flash-forwards,'" 453; Holmes, "Imagery about suicide," 431.

143 Lisa K. Libby et al., "Picture yourself at the polls: visual perspective in mental imagery affects self-perception and behavior," *Psychological Science* 18, no. 3 (March 2007): 199.

144 Holmes, "Imagery about suicide," 431.

Fortunately for Elena, she has not intended on physical harm due to her flash-forwards. The morning after that violent night, she was introduced to PMDD by a close friend and found support shortly after from another friend who is a fellow sufferer. Her friends, partner, and therapy helped to steer her quickly in a more positive direction, but, as I've discussed, finding answers and support so promptly is not the story for many women.

For some, the lack of a diagnosis or understanding can lead them to take more drastic actions, as was the case for now-thirty-seven-year-old Nicki.

***

Nicki's first nervous breakdown happened in sixth grade.

In fifth grade, her family uprooted themselves to move from the Netherlands to Colorado, forcing Nicki to leave her friends and the rest of her family behind. Finding herself isolated from everyone and everything she had grown up with, and situated in a strange environment, Nicki felt as if her life had suddenly flipped on its head. As her family struggled financially after the relocation, living primitively in a remote cabin with no indoor plumbing, Nicki struggled to cope with the mounting life stressors and lack of a support system.

On top of it all came puberty and the unknown threat of PMDD.

One night that year, the emotional pain became too much and Nicki felt she had no escape. Lying alone in her cabin, she was overwhelmed by feelings of wanting to kill herself.

Her stressors began following her to sleep. She began having vivid terror dreams of acts of violence committed against her or people she knew. Nicki was always the victim or bystander, unable to defend herself or others as the unnamed perpetrator struck again and again and again. She would wake sweaty and gasping as her panic attack crashed over her, the physical manifestation of her subconscious turbulence.

The emotional and environmental strains, the nightmares, the suicidal thoughts—everything combined led to a nervous breakdown. Nicki's head felt like it was full of loose electrical wires, sparking and crackling as she found no release or respite. All it took was one wrong move jostling the hot wires together and her brain exploded.

She finally told her mom she couldn't suffer like this anymore. She needed to get away from everything for a while and live with her grandparents. Removed from the tensions and hardships at home, Nicki hoped things would start to improve. She thought her problems were ascribed to reactions from life events and stressors, so by taking action and putting energy into better managing her life, Nicki trusted she could right her fractured mental state.

"That's why PMDD is so challenging," Nicki argues, "because we can ascribe our symptoms to life stressors, and no one sees there is another problem. Professionals and loved ones just think we don't have the ability to cope well, not understanding something else is going on."

Understandably, Nicki saw little improvement from her efforts to compartmentalize and alleviate life stressors.

The anxiety and feelings of panic didn't go away, and other symptoms such as fatigue, irritability, angry outbursts, feeling despondent, blurred vision, and a lack of spatial awareness followed.

She found herself living in the perpetual now and would struggle to recall what she had done the week or month before, unless she had written it down. Planning, writing things down, and diligently taking notes became her coping method to attempt to control and manage life.

Some days she would wake up feeling so tired and despondent all she wanted to do was stay in bed all day. But she didn't. She forced herself out of bed and through the day, even when doing so felt like a Herculean effort.

Nicki continued to believe depression, ongoing life stressors and traumatic childhood events, and her strained relationship with her mom were the culprits for her symptoms, and she personally was failing at navigating challenging situations and pressures.

> *Although not conclusive, several studies have correlated high levels of stress and trauma exposure to PMDD, so there is a possibility Nicki's history could have contributed to or exacerbated her symptoms.*[145]

---

145 Raffi and Freeman, "The etiology of premenstrual," 26; Corey E. Pilver, "Posttraumatic stress disorder and trauma characteristics are correlates of premenstrual dysphoric disorder," *Archives of Women's Mental Health* 14, no. 5 (July 2011): 383; Elizabeth R. Bertone-Johnson et al., "Early life emotional, physical, and sexual abuse and the development of premenstrual syndrome: a longitudinal study," *Journal of Women's Health* 23, no. 9 (September 2014): 737.

Yet, even after cutting negative influences out of her life and incorporating therapy and multiple lifestyle changes into her routine, Nicki's symptoms persisted.

She began to blame herself for her outbursts, panic attacks, and foggy memory. She felt like there was something wrong with her, but she didn't know what. She needed to fix it, but she didn't know how. She kept unintentionally hurting those around her, and in response they hurt her back.

Unable to control her emotions and intense reactions, it was as if there was a monster lurking in her brain she just couldn't expunge. Confused, helpless, and angry at the part of herself which seemed self-destructive, she began turning on herself too.

As her relationships with friends, family, and partners suffered and as she let people walk all over her, Nicki hit some of the lowest points of her life.

For those few weeks before her period started every month, respite and peace were rare. Finding little solace from her fractured and confused support network, Nicki's self-destructive thoughts drove her to escape the overwhelming emotional pain with the blade of a kitchen knife on multiple occasions. She often didn't realize what she was doing or would dissociate completely from her actions.

In one incident, all she had to remember it was by someone else's retelling of the event. A friend, who was present at the time, recounted it to Nicki years later.

Nicki's actions sprung from desperation and were yet another story of the medical system's failure. The first time she went to the doctor about her symptoms was as a teen during a spell of particularly bad fatigue. At the clinic, she was tested for mono and when the results came back negative, they told her she was probably depressed, chemically imbalanced, and hypoglycemic.

Throughout her twenties that continued to be the response she received from countless other doctors who either dismissed her concerns or inadequately diagnosed her. Nicki eventually took it upon herself to do her own research and track her symptoms to provide some more clarity. In her late twenties, she connected the timing of her symptoms to her period cycle, noticing they would start a week or two before she began menstruating each month.

So, she chalked it up to really bad PMS. She thought her emotional ordeals which made it nearly impossible for her to get out of bed or sent her into bouts of uncontrollable rage could be attributed to mood-influencing hormone fluctuations.

In a way, yes, PMDD is similar to a form of severe PMS. But in another way, PMDD is a whole different ball game.

> *According to David Goldman from the US National Institutes of Health, the key difference between someone who suffers from PMS and someone who suffers from PMDD is, "women with PMDD have an intrinsic difference in their molecular apparatus for response to sex hormones—not just emotional behaviors they should be able to voluntarily control."*[146]

146 Fiona McDonald, "Scientists Think They Might Have Figured Out The Cause of Severe PMS," Science Alert, January 5, 2017.

Although some of Nicki's symptoms and their timing were similar to common PMS symptoms, she was missing information about their true underlying cause.

In her early thirties she started studying to become certified as a holistic wellness coach, and as part of her training she had to carefully and thoroughly track everything going on with her body and mind. It was during that time she connected her symptoms to her changing progesterone levels and brought this new information to her current doctor.

Yet, not only was this doctor evidently unaware or uneducated on PMDD, Nicki was also unfortunately in the middle of her monthly PMDD cycle during the appointment. The doctor was quick to dismiss Nicki's concerns, informing her progesterone levels fluctuate normally throughout the month, so they couldn't possibly test to confirm her theory and sent her on her way.

The hard truth is, after more than two decades of suffering, Nicki only got a definitive and accurate diagnosis after she unwittingly put the right combination of words in her search bar and happened upon her ever-elusive condition. After learning of the existence of PMDD, finding a new doctor, and presenting that as a possible answer, Nicki got her diagnosis.

Though her treatment continues to be an uphill battle, as there is no conclusive cure or treatment for PMDD, the diagnosis itself proved a reparative force.

Armed with information and a clearer understanding of her condition, Nicki has been able to educate her family and boyfriend. She says, "For me, having a diagnosis has been such a relief and a blessing for [my family] and our relationships together. Because now, finally, we all know what it is."

That small nugget of validation and confirmation has opened up channels of communication, and Nicki has slowly grown more comfortable sharing openly about what she needs and what she's feeling with her closest family and friends.

Being able to rely on that support network again has been hugely beneficial for Nicki, and she has been able to at least manage some of her symptoms through therapy and her holistic health approaches as a wellness coach. That being said, her health and well-being journey is a continuing challenge, made more difficult by the advent of another condition in her mid-thirties known as menorrhagia.

> *Menorrhagia is the term for menstrual periods with abnormally heavy or prolonged bleeding. People who suffer from menorrhagia will often soak through one or more sanitary pads or tampons every hour for several consecutive hours, will bleed for more than a week regularly, and experience symptoms of anemia, such as fatigue or shortness of breath, due to loss of blood.*[147]

---

147 "Menorrhagia (heavy menstrual bleeding)," Mayo Clinic, accessed May 15, 2020.

Unlike Courtney and Caroline, when Nicki's period starts now, her ability to function normally does not return.

In Nicki's case, her condition puts her out for two to three days once she starts her period due to painful cramps and excessive bleeding. She can't be up and about during those days without feeling extreme dizziness or a loss of consciousness—and that's *with* medication to slow her bleeding.

Nicki likes to joke she has to "go with the flow," quite literally, as she goes from one cycle right into the next every month. Anyone who has had a period has probably, at some point, had to adjust their daily activities to accommodate for especially bad cramps, or uncomfortable bloating, or general tiredness.

But for Nicki, with PMDD and menorrhagia, she has had to largely restructure her life according to what her body needs.

For a long time, Nicki would try to push through her symptoms: when her body was telling her she was tired, she would ignore the fatigue and force herself through normal daily activities. But these habits just served to amplify her emotional symptoms, worsening her irritability and mood swings. Instead, she now tries to be more in tune and responsive to her body's needs.

Not exactly easy when you're not entirely functional for half of every month.

As women, we often receive very mixed messages when it comes to how we should operate while on our periods.

On the one hand, the popular trope for a woman on her period is characterized by irrational outbursts of anger, crying inconsolably over any ad with a dog in it, and a face full of Ben & Jerry's. It's meant to be a comedic portrayal or a brush-off rationale of behavior from women that is not balanced, calm, and pleasing.

Because god forbid women to show any distasteful emotion aside from the time of the month we are bleeding from our vaginas.

This imagery also signals all women are hot messes during their periods, playing into the sexist mindset women are too emotionally unstable to act as effective leaders, to be taken seriously, or to conduct themselves capably compared to their male counterparts.

On the other hand, women also are taught we should just be able to continue as if everything is normal when we're on our periods. This is in part a product of the normalization of female pain and in part a defense of, or rebuttal to, the aforementioned blubbering, emotional trope.

But ads like the "Play on" Playtex Tampon commercials, which features women athletes kicking ass while purportedly on their periods, are actually discouraging to someone like Nicki who physically cannot "play on" during her period.

That's not to say companies like Playtex are putting out a negative or falsifying narrative. In fact, it's meant to be empowering, showing girls and women don't have to let their "time of the month" limit what they can do. It's simply important to recognize it's also okay if you can't function as you normally would before or during your period, and that doesn't make you weaker or overly emotional.

For someone like Nicki, taking a break and restructuring how she works when she's in the midst of her back-to-back cycles was a necessity. She now practices what she calls "unconditional self-care" by being brutally honest about what she can and can't handle and focusing on her top priorities.

We need to reformat how we think and inform people about periods. Starting from when we first learn about the menstrual cycle, we need to include discussions about hormones, not just mentioning they cause the physical process to occur but, explaining how they can impact our emotions in a very real way.

We need dialogue about a range of period experiences, not just the "normal" range of experiences. This will facilitate conversations that distinguish between a healthy period with minimal side effects, and a period which results in damaging or life-threatening physical effects, thoughts, and behaviors.

Many PMDD sufferers don't realize for years their symptoms have anything to do with their period cycle because while we're taught about cramps, the emotional effects are rarely covered in depth. PMDD is a complex issue, there's no question, and it's the responsibility of our medical providers to understand the science and biology behind each sufferer's symptoms.

But also bringing the idea of PMDD into the mainstream sex ed curriculum and period discourse can point sufferers in the direction of answers, make them feel less alone in what they're going through, and quite literally save lives.

CHAPTER 8

Taking up Space

I'll invite you inside my humble home
to see the wreck I made amongst the treasures
I've collected over time.
I'll even show you my scrapbook of unconditional
friends and saucy lovers, or I'll read a few
of the hopes and losses written in the
leather journal by my bed.
I could show you my scars
and my favorite album on vinyl.
I could crack a joke to make you laugh if you prefer.
Then we can all sit down for coffee, and once you're
comfortable, maybe we can talk about the musty
opened box I've placed on the kitchen table.

—Excerpt from *Come Over* by Trista Marie McGovern[148]

***

Clad in a bright orange bikini, the straps wrapping twice
around her back and snaking up her neck, Trista fiddles
with the silver band around her thumb as she waits for the

---

148 Trista Marie McGovern, "Come Over," Instagram, February 22, 2020.

camera to click. The shutter goes and she stands to inspect the photo. Unsatisfied, she repositions the tripod so the camera can capture the spots of light falling on the dark blue wall and resets the timer.

She kneels once again on the worn wooden floor, her right arm cradling her left, her lips painted a deep burgundy, looking off solemnly at some unknown encumbrance. The photo seems to fall, following the light down the wall as it drips onto her right shoulder, casting the front of her body in sunshine and growing darker as it slips down, tracing the S-shaped curvature of her form, before arcing over the just visible lotus tattoo stamped on her left thigh and disappearing into her body's shadow.

Happy with the photo, Trista moves to take the last shot of the day. This time, she stands close to the wall with her back to the camera. Hair pinned up, a strong, white beam of light slices diagonally across the top half of the frame, hitting her back squarely on the left side. The brightest point pools in the dip of her spine, just where her left shoulder blade touches right above her hip.

Born with severe scoliosis and an underdeveloped left arm (called radial dysplasia), Trista has a C-curved spine and a club arm with four fingers. Yet, she is not the type to allow others to define her solely by her disabilities.

After finishing her photoshoot, she places a robe over the Fantabody bikini and snaps a lens cap on her camera. Later, she sends her favorite photos off to Vogue magazine where they will be featured later that month, along with an interview. It's part of Fantabody's Fantagirl project which

promotes embracing diversity by encouraging every partic-
ipant to portray her seductive uniqueness in an effort to start
conversations around disability, immigration, and sex work.

The shots Trista chose of herself are intentionally powerful and vulnerable—the culmination of a year filled with
finally openly recognizing her body and the sexual being
hidden inside.

***

There was a point in her life when she could never have put
herself on display so publicly. Growing up in a small town
in Wisconsin, Trista was more focused on blending in than
standing out. She never allowed her disability to interfere
with her life, and never made excuses or bowed down to any
challenges. Even while facing multiple surgeries for her scoliosis, or missing class due to her weakened immune system,
Trista always managed to remain positive and never dwelled
on the obstacles life drew up for her.

"I always tried to do the same things as everyone else because
I didn't like to draw attention to myself," she recalls. "I'd find
ways to adapt."[149]

As a visibly disabled person, Trista says there is a tendency
to always be hyper aware of her body and what other people
think of her—what she looks like, how she acts, what she
says. Tiptoeing around her disabilities as a young girl, and

---

149 Autumn Grooms, "Extra Effort: Tomah's Trista McGovern accepts
every challenge, is a role model," *La Crosse Tribune*, March 19, 2011.

especially as an adolescent, she tried to ignore them in hopes others would begin to ignore them too.

She made it a habit to shut out the parts of herself that might make others uncomfortable. At the lunch table, as her girlfriends sat around giggling about their crushes or which jock was the hottest that year, Trista kept her mouth shut. No matter she also thought those boys were cute—she was sure voicing that particular opinion would shift the mood because her friends would think it was weird or awkward that she had those thoughts, too.

So, she kept those feelings tamped down. She didn't see sexuality being represented within the context of disability, and for years she largely avoided anything to do with attraction or dating, or at least stayed private about her experiences.

It didn't help her sex ed classes at school were more focused on scare tactics than anything else. She remembers they talked about STIs and how you can get pregnant and somebody threw up once from a series of disturbing photos of infected genitalia.

"But there was never anything about different bodies, or trans, or even just pleasure or consent," she says. "There was no defining what assault is or any of the above. It's always just like, you'll get STIs, just so you know. That's it."

It wasn't until much later when Trista realized her sex ed had left her with large gaps.

College brought with it a more open environment for her to experiment with dating. post-grad, she became involved in disability justice, which opened her eyes to ableism, a lack of disability representation, and an absence of space for disabled people within the realm of sexuality. Trista realized for most of her life, she had not been at the table when it came to talking about disability rights. For most of her life, many of the messages she received seemed to suggest disability was not something people wanted to talk about or hear about, so she had actively avoided the topic.

"How are we supposed to put ourselves in the conversation when we're left in the other room?" Trista asks, "How do we get and/or feel invited to the circle when we seem covered in red flags? How can we rectify the twisted connotation that disabled means nonsexual when you perpetuate it? How can we process our layers of trauma when we're too busy putting you at ease? How do we put ourselves out there when people with disabilities are three times more likely to be sexually assaulted than literally anyone else? How can we expect healthy relationships when you'll either love us or fuck us, but rarely both?"[150]

Trista points out a striking dichotomy here, one in which able-bodied individuals tend to view disabled individuals as childish and asexual, while at the same time seeing them as easily taken advantage of, objectified, or tokenized. Disabled people are often not perceived as having bodily autonomy or as having the mental wherewithal to make and hold adult desires and choices.

---

150 Trista Marie McGovern, "Dismantling What We've Been Told About Disability and Sexuality," The Mighty, December 27, 2019.

Instead they are viewed as objects—to play with, to preserve, to get inspiration from, to discard. It's an issue of infantilization which seeps into every aspect of their life.

Like when they are talked down to like children because they're seen as cognitively impaired or sub-human due to bodily differences.

Or, when they are not afforded the right to adult habits and behaviors because they're expected to be naive and pure.

Ignored. Censored. Stifled.

Infantilizing people with physical disabilities removes them from conversations about their bodies and their lives, sticking them in a state of limbo as able-bodied people around them are free to grow and mature and express themselves as they please.

Trista describes it like a snowball effect. People don't talk about the intersection of disability and sexuality because it is seen as a personal issue, or too complicated, or too uncomfortable, and so it's never tackled in sex ed, in general conversation, or in the media.

"And then that just escalates because it's not talked about," she argues, "and since it's not talked about, people with disabilities feel like they can't be at the table for the conversation. Then other people at the table are leaving them out of the conversation because they're not at the table and they never have to think about it. It just keeps getting worse when the lack of representation ends up making people with disabilities feel like they truly don't belong."

This snowball effect quickly grows into internalized ableism which can really impact anyone who does not fit the able-bodied "norm." For Trista, who is especially visibly disabled, she felt as if she constantly had to manage other people's reactions and emotions to her body based on their presumptions about her disability. She learned to prioritize and ensure other people felt comfortable in her presence, instead of honoring her own needs, feelings, and emotions first.

Discussing sexuality, even to talk about crushes or dating, was definitely not a topic she felt she could broach. That would require her to unpack everything from internalized ableism to dealing with people's reactions to her unpacking internalized ableism to realizing this is more than a personal obstacle; it's a systemic political issue.

Trista argues, "sexuality just happens to be the most neglected and 'controversial' facet; in turn, being sexual in a visually disabled body feels like protesting...Disability is the largest minority, and the only one that can suddenly become an attribute to anyone at any point in their life. But it seems to be the one talked about the least, sexuality being the least discussed topic. I've seen persons with disabilities and/or visible difference as either objects to be examined or as tokens for inspiration, but never just as humans within the umbrella of sexuality."[151]

When Trista finally found herself in a space mentally where she could, bit by bit, push herself out of her comfort zone

---

151   McGovern, "Come Over"; McGovern, "Dismantling."

and face those twisted, deeply rooted messages, she describes feeling like she was "just ripping off all the band aids."

Her love of photography and poetry guided her as she started to explore themes of sexuality and body positivity, and she gradually found her voice through this creative avenue. She started shooting her friends and models, often flung over beds, scantily clad or tastefully nude. More often than not brazenly staring down the camera, her models seem comfortable and self-assured, daring you to say something. She captures the whole, as well as pieces: a leg here, a hip there, a tattoo, and many, many hands.

"With my high value and gravitation toward empathy, the human condition, and connection, one of my largest amounts of work includes intimate portraits," Trista says. "With a great fondness for people, my work of portraits is created with focusing on breaking down barriers to illuminate vulnerability and individual personalities. Therefore, the photos often have minimal clothing and environments, with all facades of expressions removed to help represent the honest, raw human at hand."

It wasn't until a few years later Trista began to explore her own body through photography, capturing her bare back covered in flowers, or a glimpse of her thigh sporting her lotus flower tattoo.

She had never let people photograph her before; she was always the one behind the camera. Safe and in control.

But slowly, she began to publicly post more and more photos of her body, growing more confident, and realizing her posts were resonating with people. It was uncomfortable to post the photos at first, even though she expected generally positive reactions.

What she didn't foresee was the outpouring of support from thousands of new followers.

"I expected it to just have a bunch of likes and like, 'Go you, good job Trista!' But it was so much more than I thought it was going to be. I was actually kind of shocked there was such a reaction to it, so that was really impactful for me. But there were also so many people who reached out and said they just bawled. Because they felt heard."

Trista realized these conversations needed to be had, and about a year and a half ago she decided to start writing about it, with visuals to complement the messages of sexuality and disability.

"I knew if I just wrote, people wouldn't read it. They wouldn't. It's easier when you can put a face to the words and then the words are extra and it gives us the story, and the explanation of the issues."

In these photos, though, she wouldn't be alone. And she was very particular about who she chose for her first series.

***

The day of the shoot, the only people in the room were Trista, the photographer, and Trista's friend Brian.

Brian fits society's typical standard for attractiveness: an able-bodied, tall, white, conventionally good-looking guy. Positioning him in photos where he is stroking Trista's bare back or enveloping her small frame or in bed with their hands next to one another's are powerful contrasts: it's not what people expect or are used to seeing depicted.

"Just having him in a photo with me where it suggests intimacy is visually jarring for people," explains Trista.

She had hesitated to do this for a long time because she knew she had to go about it in a tactful way. She didn't want pity, she didn't want to be an "inspiration," she just wanted the conversation to happen.

She was a little nervous, too.

As Trista climbed onto the bed, a nervous tremor tickled her spine from her body telling her she shouldn't be doing this. She felt ready and determined, but even now Trista still feels uncomfortable being photographed.

She couldn't help feeling awkward about being on display in her most vulnerable state. Most anyone would.

But it's especially difficult for someone who has had to live with deeply rooted internalized messages which promote able bodies as the ideal for beauty and ignore any bodies that look different. It can be difficult to dispel those negative messages and feel sexy and beautiful in front of the unforgiving lens of a camera.

"I'm not a model," she laughs, "You know people call me that. I mean, technically, I guess I am. But it's hard to accept, and it's weird to think about."

Trista may not think of herself that way, but her modeling is breaking into a space rarely touched but desperately in need of attention. She considers herself lucky because she's not shy or introverted, and she's not afraid to be as "obnoxious" (as she puts it) as she pleases about disability justice.

It's all paid off. Her first photo essay series almost immediately went viral, and following several other shoots, including Vogue, she has gained over thirty thousand followers on Instagram. People connect to her vulnerability and her words, especially those who have never seen a body like theirs represented in such a beautiful, sensual way or have their tumultuous inner thoughts put into such striking words.

"Despite my continual contradictory opinion on publicly broadcasting that secret box under the floorboards and putting my ass on the stage with full expectations of awkward scrutiny, I believe taking up space can be a beautiful necessary evil," she stresses.[152]

But it was, and still is, a process to get to the place and headspace she is in today where she can post about her issues and actually feel good about it. For a long time, as she was dealing with unpacking her disability and her internalized ableism, as well as inevitable life traumas and dramas, she had to put a large part of her sexuality on the back burner.

---

152 Ibid.

Traversing the complicated societal fabric of sexuality as a queer person is difficult enough with an able body, but it was not a top priority to explore that part of herself when she was just beginning to openly embrace her dating life and when she was just beginning to see herself as a person who could even be part of the sexuality conversation.

To leave that side of herself out of the picture, though, would be to erase an essential part of herself. Several months after her photo series with Brian, she posted another, this time with a lanky brunette woman straddling her, embracing her, holding her. It's stunning and sensual and audacious. It's a spectacle simply because it's intimate and vulnerable and not normalized.

It's a spectacle, but it shouldn't have to be.

"I've found it's nearly impossible to separate my own precious intricate personal life from the words that need to be swallowed and eventually settled into the spines of everyone else."[153]

It has to be shoved in people's faces according to Trista, otherwise visibility of these issues will never gain traction. But it's important to remember, too, the toll it can take on the person shouldering the responsibility of dusting up all the crap continuously swept under the rug.

Trista has come so far in her personal journey, from avoidance to acceptance to advocacy. The camera shows her as

---

153 Ibid.

happy and confident, for the most part accurately mirroring her life full of amazing friends, a successful photography career, and healthy body normalization.

But she describes posting as a sort of high-followed-by-a-hangover experience. There's an initial rush when she starts getting likes and followers and knows it's reaching more and more people, but the next day she can't help wishing her posts didn't always have to blow up with such a reaction, be it positive or negative.

"It reaches people so much because it's not normalized," she argues, "and it's because I'm different and because it's something new to people. So, the next day I always feel like, 'Oh, this is stupid.' It shouldn't be that inspirational, it shouldn't be so moving because it should just be normal, but it's not."

It's a lot to put yourself out there so honestly and openly for thousands of people to see, and moreover, to feel as if your vulnerability is responsible for a larger movement—a movement impacting the largest minority group in the US.

In reality, a lot of the responsibility to shift away from normalizing abled bodies and "othering" disabled bodies falls on able-bodied people to make space in media representation, popular culture, and general conversation for disabled people to speak their truths. This means for people like Trista who want to be public about their sexuality, we have to be conscious about celebrating her narrative and not sensationalizing it. We have to remember hers is just one story, and women with disabilities exist on the spectrum of sexuality and sexual openness just as any able-bodied woman does.

Falling into or remaining comfortable with erroneous stereotypes about disability and sexuality can be incredibly damaging to someone's self-image and relationship with their body and can have broader implications for someone's ability to access sexual health care, as we'll explore further in the next chapter.

CHAPTER 9

Infantilized or Fetishized: The Unfortunate Paradox

Her phone dinged and Elizabeth snatched it from the counter, eager to read the reply. She'd met the guy online and after hitting it off over text, she suggested they meet up in person tomorrow night for drinks. There was a cute bar down the street she had been dying to try out. Opening her lock screen, his response glared back at her.

"Wait, do you have a disability?"

Pausing in confusion, Elizabeth left the message on read as she logged onto her online dating profile, just to make sure she wasn't going crazy.

Scrolling through her bio, her eyes landed on the evidence: the words *Paralympic swimmer* plainly written. She snorted. They had been chatting for *weeks*, had he really just put two and two together?

Why did it suddenly matter?

Returning to her messages, she quipped back, "Ya, last I checked." She was met with radio silence.

That is, until he deigned to reply a few days later with, "Ya, I can't deal with that." As if when the security of the screen barrier was just about to disappear, her body became too uncomfortable for him to handle.

Born with limb difference, Elizabeth is all too familiar with the stigmas, stereotypes, and biases able-bodied people have regarding bodies that stray from the "norm." With a shortened right arm and a prosthetic right leg, Elizabeth is very aware sometimes her visible disability is all people see when they look at her.

But contrary to popular able-bodied notions, she never allows her disability to act as a limitation. Winning her first medal at the 1996 Atlanta Paralympic Games when she was just sixteen, and then two more at the Sydney games four years later, Elizabeth had already proved herself an international powerhouse at the tender age of twenty.

Surrounded by others with disabilities—friends, teammates, opponents—Elizabeth had spent most of her adolescence ensconced in a community of disabled athletes. Her Paralympic status meant she never had a typical teenage experience, and it also meant she spent many of her formative years protected from the acute discovery and realization of disability discrimination.

It wasn't until she retired from swimming at the age of twenty-one and entered the university where she truly encountered the idea of disability injustice, amassing vocabulary and knowledge of previously unfamiliar concepts like "disability politics" and "disability activism" through her studies in fine arts.

"I think it opened up my eyes to the discrimination disabled people, myself included, were going through on a daily basis which I'd never actually recognized. I felt like I'd had a hood over my head for all of my life and then suddenly this hood was pulled back and I could see what was actually going on around me," she explains.

Elizabeth began to pick up on micro-aggressions and displays of ableism in her day-to-day life.

As an employee at the post office, she was once patted on the hand and called a "clever darling" because she, a full-fledged adult, successfully deposited **and** withdrew money for a customer.[154]

While gathering supplies from a farm equipment shop for a college class project, she was flat-out ignored by a salesperson who thought it made more sense to ask her father about the materials needed for the installation art piece *Elizabeth* was creating.[155]

She was no stranger to the often humiliating, frustrating, patronizing infantilization of her person.

---

154 Elizabeth Wright, "Infantilising Disabled People is a Thing and You're Probably Unconsciously Doing It," Medium, January 13, 2020.

155 Ibid.

It bleeds into almost every aspect of her life:

- in baby talk
- in being passed over in favor of only addressing an able-bodied person
- and in the assumption being disabled is tantamount to being asexual.

"I think the biggest myth about disability and sexuality, especially around disabled women, is asexuality," she states. "People believe you mustn't want to have sex. You mustn't have relationships with people; you just can't be interested in that."

This narrative does not only come from potential romantic partners, like the guy who couldn't seem to grasp the meaning behind the words *Paralympic* and *prosthetic*.

Elizabeth remembers an incident a few months back involving her housemate, we'll call her Amy, and some friends. At the time, Elizabeth and Amy had been living together for about four years and were quite good friends. Over the years, Elizabeth had met many of Amy's friends and formed her own friendships with several of them.

One day Amy was out with some mutual friends without Elizabeth, and they began discussing disability and sexuality, which quickly led to Amy's friends prying into Elizabeth's romantic life. They needled Amy with questions, asking things like:

"Has Elizabeth ever had a boyfriend?"

"Has she ever had sex?"

"Has she ever done this? Has she ever done that?"

When Amy divulged the conversation to her housemate, Elizabeth's first thought was *Why did they ask Amy? Wouldn't I know the answers to these questions better?*

She wondered from where this piqued curiosity and fascination came.

Was she a spectacle at which to marvel?

An object at which to poke and prod and wonder?

"They were believing stereotypes from disability narratives that are entrenched in society and that are blatantly not true," she says. They were not just believing them, but actively spreading them about someone for whom they know and care.

But it's just as Trista says, "you'll either love us or fuck us but rarely both," because just as there is a tendency to view and treat people who are disabled as children, as naive and pure, there is also a tendency at the other end of the spectrum to hyper-sexualize and fetishize disabled bodies.

***

After college, Elizabeth faced the big life question all grads must confront once propelled out of those ivy-clad brick walls: what now?

Her whole life, before attending the university, had been consumed by her swimming career: training and traveling and competing. Now she had a master's degree, a whole world of possibilities, and a background to leverage.

She began public speaking in schools, starting out as an inspirational speaker before realizing the majority of the questions she got after she finished telling her audience about her Paralympic journey were centered around her disability, rather than being centered around her sport.

Her interest in disability justice, which had blossomed during her time at the university, slowly pushed itself into the limelight as Elizabeth realized these kids wanted to know more, and should know more, in the name of spreading disability awareness and allyship. Continuing her public speaking and guest lecturing, she began centering her messages around disability inclusion and started a publication called *Conscious Being* on Medium dedicated to sharing the stories and voices of other disabled women.

But it was her YouTube channel which first exposed her directly to a darker side of disability support groups.

***

The message seemed harmless enough: "I really like your videos."

The comment was nestled among many other positive comments posted under Elizabeth's latest upload, a video showing how she painted her fingernails on her left hand with her shortened right arm. But, when a few days later the same user asked her to do a video where she painted the toenails on her prosthetic leg, Elizabeth started to feel uneasy.

After digging a little deeper, she found hundreds of liked videos under his account of limb different people and amputees—vlogging, doing mundane tasks, suggestively removing their prosthetic legs.

The list went on.

Elizabeth had stumbled upon one of the members of a fetish group known as devotees.

> *A devotee is someone sexually attracted to or aroused by disabled people and their struggles.*[156]

This was not the first time she had heard of this group. A master's student at one of her guest lectures, an above-knee amputee, introduced Elizabeth to the fetish group, including some of the more terrifying sides of their devotion such as stalking and physical and emotional abuse. Now, Elizabeth shuddered to think what was happening behind computer screens at the expense of her videos meant for children.

At the expense of her own personal integrity.

Elizabeth argues devotee-ism is "a special form of objectification and fetishization that doesn't get talked about often.

---

156 Emily Yates, "'Pretty Cripples' and the people turned on by disability," BBC, March 12, 2016.

But it has to be talked about. It has to emerge from the murky undergrowth of sexual harassment and sexual abuse. It has to be confronted for its problematic attitude toward disabled people."[157]

And she's right. Because at its heart, it is objectification of a body. It is seeing a person as a sum of pleasing body parts which exist for someone else's sexual pleasure, whether consensual or not.

In particular, the issue of devotee-ism differs in comparison to other non-consensual objectification able-bodied women confront due to the unfortunate social reality within which disabled women reside. The truth of the matter is their devotion can quickly turn threatening or perverted when the fetishizer feels entitled to the woman's body *because* she is disabled or believes her to be "weaker [and] easier to control and manipulate."[158]

Of course, as is common, there are two sides to every coin. Some devotees do respect boundaries and are hyper-aware their group can make disabled people feel uncomfortable. They may even try to encourage other members to tone down the creepy.

Also, there are disabled people who do willingly engage with devotees. Sometimes this can be for sensual purposes to feel sexier in their own bodies. Sometimes the relationships are more transactional, exchanging photos for money

---

157 Elizabeth Wright, "Devoted to Disability: are devotees really that creepy?" Medium, May 6, 2020.
158 Ibid.

in a purely platonic and professional manner. *The crucial difference with these interactions is they are completely on the disabled person's terms, they benefit both parties, and leave the disabled person with control over their bodily autonomy.*

But Elizabeth is not yet ready to indulge her devotees. When she gets DMs on her social media accounts, she quickly blocks them. Many devotees are quick to ridicule the so-called "haters," or those in the disabled community who don't want their attention. Devotees think they're just showing disability extra love, so disabled people should be thankful in return. But disabled bodies are not anyone's to control or discard., to dictate or ignore, or to love or detest.

As Lara Clarke, a contributor to the *Conscious Being* publication highlights in her experience as a disabled woman: "Apparently, my choices are a) wheel the streets un-harassed, safe in the knowledge that society will never view me as a fully-functioning, fully sexual human being, or b) live in constant fear of verbal taunts, groping and worse because at least that would mean I'd passed some kind of societal attractiveness test."[159]

Why does it have to be one or the other?

Infantilized or sexualized.

Unsexy or fetishistic.

---

159   Lara Clarke, "I've Never Been Catcalled, and I Don't Know How to Feel about it," Medium, April 23, 2020.

What Elizabeth wants is not to be seen as her disability, but to be seen as a person. A person who has hopes and dreams and goals. A person who curses and drinks and has sex. A person deserving of respect and independence and love.

***

Elizabeth is not her disability, but that doesn't mean her disability isn't important. Especially when it comes to her sexual health, recognizing and understanding her disability is something she wishes her doctors did more.

Unsurprisingly, she has faced a medical milieu which is dismissive at worst and uncomfortable at best. She has experienced first-hand what happens when the false narratives surrounding disabled people seep into the health arena—namely when her doctors in the past assumed Elizabeth wasn't having sex and therefore, never insisted she get a Pap smear.

Even when Elizabeth explicitly asked to go on the pill, she says her doctor still did not logically connect, or even ask, if she wanted birth control because she was having unprotected sex. This is particularly worrying in Elizabeth's case, as both her mom and her aunt died from womb cancer.

Finding a provider who actually listened to her concerns and treated her like a woman, not a child, was not the end of Elizabeth's problems at the doctor's office. Physically getting a Pap smear proved to be a whole other ordeal, and a painful process overall. To successfully maneuver into the correct position with her shortened right leg is a hassle and very uncomfortable for her hip bone to hold during the test.

"I think in terms of sexual health there has to be more of an understanding of the body—and differences in the body—that might make a procedure more uncomfortable, even impossible for some people," Elizabeth says. "It's just not completely accessible at the moment to every single woman. Is there not a way doctors can work with the disabled patients to actually figure out how to make tests or procedures more accessible to disabled women instead of just having flat denial of, 'Oh they're probably not having sex,' or, 'We physically can't do this.' When actually, perhaps, if you speak to the disabled person and work with them you could figure out a way they could have these tests done."

The health system has an obligation to provide inclusive services which cater to the needs of abled bodies and treat disabled people as whole human beings with the right to information on sexual and reproductive health. A lack of disability inclusion leaves the population vulnerable to health risks and denies them resources readily available to abled bodies.[160]

Despite the fact 26 percent of adults in the US have some type of disability, health care barriers to the community are still extremely prevalent.[161] According to a study conducted by the Association of University Centers on Disabilities (AUCD), though more than half of women with disabilities wanted information from their doctor about sexuality, less than

---

160 Tanisha Clarke, "Disability Rights and Sexual Health," Association of Maternal & Child Health Programs, accessed June 16, 2020.

161 "Disability Impacts All of Us," Centers for Disease Control and Prevention, accessed June 22, 2020.

20 percent of their providers offered the information.[162] In another study, nearly one-third of physically disabled women reported being denied access to care from a medical provider because of their disability.[163]

Many of these barriers exist because of wrongful assumptions from health care providers that being disabled correlates to being sexually inactive, and paternalistic judgments about a disabled person's capacity to consent to or have sexual experiences.[164] Additionally, a lack of understanding or familiarity with physical or communicative adjustments that may need to be incorporated, such as lengthier appointment times or exam accommodations for patients who may be limb different or who can't stand, contributes to unequal access to quality health care.[165]

As a result, women with disabilities are less likely to receive regular preventative sexual health services, including:

- birth control
- Pap smears

162 American College of Obstetricians and Gynecologists, "Reproductive Health Care for Women With Disabilities," (Powerpoint Presentation, 2010).

163 Association of State and Territorial Health Officials, *Access to Preventive Healthcare Services for Women with Disabilities* (Arlington, VA: Association of State and Territorial Health Officials, 2013), 2, accessed June 22, 2020.

164 Anita Silvers, Leslie Francis, and Brittany Badesch, "Reproductive Rights and Access to Reproductive Services for Women with Disabilities," *American Medical Association Journal of Ethics* 18, no. 4 (April 2016): 431; Alexander Boni-Saenz, "Sexuality and Incapacity," *IIT Chicago-Kent College of Law* 76, no. 6 (September 2015): 1227.

165 Silvers et al., "Reproductive Rights," 432; Mary Ann McColl et al., "Physician Experiences Providing Primary Care to People with Disabilities," *Healthcare Policy* 4, no. 1 (August 2008): 140, 144-145.

- mammograms
- STI screenings
- and information about safe sex practices and sexual abuse resources.[166]

Women with disabilities also face the additional barrier of accessing affordable health care compared to able-bodied women. Disabled women are less likely to have private insurance, and some health care providers will refuse to treat patients without private insurance.[167] Yet, even when controlling for factors like socioeconomic status which may affect insurance coverage, adults with disabilities—women in particular—have less access to health care services.[168]

So often, in the medical field or just in general, women with disabilities are not part of the conversation. They are not asked for their input, and they are too easily ignored out of convenience. They are, as Trista mentions, not at the table.

---

166 Silvers et al., "Reproductive Rights," 432; Lisa I. Iezzoni, Stephen G. Kurtz, and Sowmya R. Rao, "Trends in Mammography Over Time for Women With and Without Chronic Disability," *Journal of Women's Health* 24, no. 7 (July 2015): 593; Lisa I. Iezzoni, Stephen G. Kurtz, and Sowmya R. Rao, "Trends in Pap Testing Over Time for Women With and Without Chronic Disability," *American Journal of Preventative Medicine* 50, no. 2 (February 2016): 210; Willi Horner-Johnson et al., "Breast and cervical cancer screening disparities associated with disability severity," *Women's Health Issues* 24, no. 1 (January 2014): 147; American College of Obstetricians and Gynecologists, "Reproductive Health."

167 Association of State and Territorial Health Officials, *Access to Preventive*, 2.

168 Silvers et al., "Reproductive Rights," 430; Elham Mahmoudi and Michelle A. Meade, "Disparities in access to health care among adults with physical disabilities: analysis of a representative national sample for a ten-year period," *Disability and Health Journal* 8, no. 2 (April 2015): 182.

But buying into stereotypes and not believing their specific lived experiences and hurdles silences them.

Promote their voices.

Break apart those horrendously inaccurate judgments.

Normalize their right to sex positivity and sexual health.

The steps we can take collectively to stop infantilizing people with disabilities and treat them like human beings rather than objects seem like common sense. But it's important for able-bodied people to always be aware of how their seemingly innocuous comments or flippant demeanor can continue to diminish disabled voices and autonomy.

The easiest thing to do is to simply treat disabled people like anyone else. When you meet them, shake their hand, make eye contact, address them directly—not an able-bodied person they are with as if they can't speak for themselves—and don't assume the able-bodied person is their caretaker. Don't use baby talk or simplify your language or ask prying and inappropriate questions.

Their bodies do not exist for your entertainment and curiosity.

"Don't reduce the disabled person to their disability," Elizabeth writes. "Being disabled is just one aspect of the human lived experience, and as actualised human beings, disabled people live as full lives as able bodied people do."[169]

---

169 Wright, "Infantilising."

This doesn't mean you should ignore the disability or minimize the challenges that come along with it. You shouldn't ignore the accommodations they may have to make in their daily life, their sex life, or their specific medical needs. But we also shouldn't view these accommodations as insurmountable obstacles.

Disability does not equal a lack of sexual desire or a lack of a healthy sex life, and contrary to popular belief, able-bodied people are not the gatekeepers of disabled people's sexualities.

CHAPTER 10

It Starts with "Hello"

Arguably, within the realm of women's and individuals assigned female at birth's sexual health, one area which remains particularly elusive to many medical practitioners is transgender health. Just ten years ago, there was no standard information about care for LGBTQ+ people, and the gap in education of health issues and care needs for this community continues to persist today.[170]

The lack of core competency training in the area of LGBTQ+ health care for future medical providers threatens the availability of affirmative care and welcoming environments for all patients.[171] As a result, transgender people confront unique barriers to adequate health care including:

- insurance coverage
- discrimination or mistreatment by health care providers

---

170 Alex S. Keuroghlian, Kevin L. Ard, and Harvey J. Makadon, "Advancing health equity for lesbian, gay, bisexual and transgender (LGBT) people through sexual health education and LGBT-affirming health care environments," *Sexual Health* 14, (February 2017): 119.

171 Ibid.

- and a lack of experience in treating trans patients on the part of health care providers.[172]

According to a 2015 National Transgender Discrimination Survey (NTDS) study, 25 percent of respondents in the past year experienced a problem with their insurance coverage related to being transgender, while 33 percent of respondents had at least one negative experience with a health care provider in the past year related to being transgender.[173]

As a trans man, Morgan Givens has experienced many of these issues. Once he started taking testosterone supplements and his outward physical appearance began to emulate his male identity, Morgan soon discovered the medical field likes to place people in boxes.

If doctors can't put a tidy little tick mark into one of the boxes on their copious patient forms, they are often at a loss.

In Morgan's case, his former physicians did not receive training in how to appropriately treat non-cisgender identities according to their specific needs and did not take the time to educate themselves retroactively even when they had trans clientele. In one instance, Morgan's doctor asked him how much testosterone he should be prescribing because the doctor was wholly unprepared to handle trans health.

Morgan was rightfully appalled.

---

172 Sandy E. James et al., *The Report of the 2015 U.S. Transgender Survey* (Washington, DC: National Center for Transgender Equality, 2016): 93, 95, 98, accessed June 8, 2020.

173 James et al., *The Report of the 2015*, 3, 95.

"Why am I teaching you to do your job?" he wondered.

This disturbing exchange with his former doctor shows not only a lack of awareness and ability to do his job inclusive of all his patients, but also highlights a lack of concern for the validity of trans health needs. He clearly did not view Morgan's testosterone levels as an important part of Morgan's overall health plan and tried to skate by on ignorance at the expense of his patient.

I have discussed in depth the issue of doctors not recognizing or believing women's sexual health concerns, but trans men and other trans people assigned female at birth face additional obstacles in this arena. It's not uncommon, for example, for trans men who are "read," or present as male but who were born with female genitalia, to not receive proper care for their bodies because of how their medical practitioners perceive them.

> *Being "read" can either mean a trans person is being read as the gender they identify as or that they are being read as cisgender. The term "read" is generally preferred to the term "passing," which is seen as implying that one should want to look cisgender, or that to be "passing" is to be "mistaken for," and therefore perpetuates the myth that trans people are deceivers.*[174]

---

174 Dawn Ennis, "10 Words Transgender People Want You to Know (But Not Say)," Advocate, February 4, 2016; "Trans 101: Glossary of Trans Words and How to Use Them," Gender Minorities, accessed October 3, 2020; "Gender Diversity Terminology," Penn State Student Affairs, accessed October 3, 2020.

When Morgan began transitioning, he started on testosterone supplements which altered his hormones to align his physical appearance with a more masculine form. But he did not have a hysterectomy and still retained the female genitalia with which he was born. His masculine outward appearance caused him to not be given the proper sexual health care for his body, like regular Pap smears, because the medical practice was holding on to a very narrow scope of gender identity and biological sex.

Equating gender and sex meant when Morgan began experiencing intense back pain and brought up concerns of ovarian cancer, as his mom had been a sufferer, he was not taken seriously.

Equating the two meant Morgan's body didn't fit their definition and was easier to ignore.

Moreover, as a black person, Morgan is not just fighting a system which actively discriminates against trans people, but one rooted in institutional racism which discounts the medical needs of people of color and further denies him access to appropriate resources and treatment.[175]

"It's exhausting to have to validate yourself constantly," Morgan says, "and then I worry about the people who are trans or queer who don't have that energy. What happens then? Where do they go when they get turned away?"

---

175 Tris Mamone, "For Trans Men Seeking Reproductive Health Care, 'There Are Barriers Every Step of the Way'," *Rewire.News*, July 3, 2019.

Trans people are not more complex or more difficult to deal with than cisgendered people. They are full humans just like anyone else, who can and should be treated in the medical field just like anyone else. AFAB trans people who have vaginas, uteruses, ovaries and menstrual cycles should be as much in the conversation about reproductive and sexual health as cis women.

But it's not as easy as just acknowledging this, and it's not something the medical community can do alone. The discrimination trans people face daily which can translate into harmful or life-threatening errors at the hands of health care providers is a product of deep-seated stigmas against the trans community.

From the continued excusal of blatant violence against trans people to the undertones of dismissal from that one aunt who can never seem to get the "confusing new pronouns" right, we constantly receive signals trans people are "wrong" or looking for attention or creepy perverts. Consequently, they face unimaginable discrimination which presents barriers at every turn, whether it be income and unemployment, violence and sexual assault, or psychological health, just to name a few.

According to a 2015 survey study conducted by the National Center for Transgender Equality:

- More than twice as many trans people live in poverty than the general US population
- The unemployment rate for trans people is three times higher than the general population
- Nearly half (47 percent) of trans respondents had been sexually assaulted in their lifetime

- 40 percent of trans respondents had attempted suicide in their lifetime (nearly nine times the rate of the general US population).[176]

Furthermore, "transgender people of color experience deeper and broader patterns of discrimination than white respondents and the U.S. population," as well as respondents with disabilities, for all of the above stats.[177]

For Morgan, it was the stories accompanying these daunting stats—depicting trans lives as dismal and full of abuse and hate—which terrorized his thoughts growing up.

He says he always knew deep down somewhere he wasn't a girl. He knew before he started puberty. He knew before he had the words to express his feelings.

What he didn't know was how his family and the world would react.

***

The first time Morgan realized there were other people out there who felt like he did was around fourth or fifth grade.

He and his brother were at their grandma's house watching TV when their programming cut to commercial break and Oprah's face appeared, her hair big and her earrings bigger. (It was the 90s, after all).

---

176 James et al., *The Report of the 2015*, 3.

177 James et al., *The Report of the 2015*, 4.

Overlaying a jazzy interlude came Oprah's voice: "On the next *Oprah Winfrey Show*, we're going to talk to families with kids who say they were born in the wrong bodies."

It was the 90s, and the terminology was off, and the tone was sensationalistic, but it clicked instantly for Morgan, who sat up so fast he nearly gave himself whiplash.

From the kitchen, his mom called out, "What are you watching out there?" before coming to investigate.

"Oh no," she exclaimed, "No, no, no. Where's the remote? You shouldn't be watching this—wouldn't want you kids to get confused, thinking there's something wrong with you. We don't have people like that in our family."

Fishing the remote from between the couch cushions, she turned the screen black, warding off those strange and potentially corrupting ideas.

In the same day, Morgan learned he wasn't alone, there were others out there like him, while also discovering his family loved him conditionally. But it was okay, because he could take his newfound awareness and just pretend, right?

Well, he could pretend until the monster named puberty reared its ugly head.

For most any kid, puberty is a wholly uncomfortable, extremely awkward inconvenience. For Morgan, it felt like his body was betraying him. It hit him like a semi, and he would spend hours in front of the mirror just roving his eyes over his new body, his new face, utterly deceived.

"I was flummoxed and perplexed my body would have the audacity to do something I didn't want it to," he recalls.

Morgan never felt hatred toward his body, but his new developments forced him to confront his feelings about his gender identity—an immensely difficult thing to do when you fear rejection from your family, friends, or society.

At the time of Morgan's adolescence, he was largely surrounded by a single trans narrative: to be trans was to be doomed.

Popular culture either left the trans community out completely, or grossly misrepresented them with inappropriate and transphobic archetypes, like serial killer "Buffalo Bill" who wears the skin of his female victims because of his "strange urges" to become a woman himself.

Morgan grew up with a media which tended to sensationalize and exaggerate trans stories, demonize trans people, and represent them in damaging ways. He overwhelmingly saw accounts of abuse, AIDS, hate crimes, homelessness, etc., with no positive stories or trans role models.

All the articles and journals and anecdotes were saying the same thing: "You are transgender, and you will die alone.

You are transgender and you will lose your home. You are transgender and no one will ever love you."[178]

Morgan became increasingly afraid of being ostracized by his family and community, but at the same time, how could he go on pretending in this new, traitorous body?

Living what felt like a lie with no positive end in sight, Morgan grew depressive and his thoughts turned suicidal.

One day, researching trans stories for the thousandth time, he happened upon an article with a phrase which struck fear and despair through his heart: trans panic.

His eyes skimmed worriedly, hurriedly, over the words which told him if he went on a date with someone and they found out he was transgender, then killed him in a moment of hate-filled, rage-filled violence, they could use gay/trans panic as a legitimate defense. They could blame their murderous actions on the gender or sexual identity of their victim, and all the police and all the jurors and all the judges would nod their heads in lawful agreement.

> *Trans panic practiced as a legally sanctioned form of discrimination is still very much in effect, with only eight states having passed bans on its use as of 2019.*[179]

---

178 *Story District*, "Morgan Givens in Story District's Emotional Overload on August 11, 2015," September 8, 2015, video, 9:58.

179 Alexandra Holden, "The Gay/Trans Panic Defense: What It is, and How to End It," American Bar Association, April 1, 2020.

It was at this moment, Morgan snapped. The decision to end his life was instantaneous.

Driven to this conclusion after weeks and months and years of desperation because he was told over and over, he couldn't find happiness since his sex and his gender didn't line up. So, with no other way out, he swallowed his carefully researched poison of choice and waited for unconsciousness to sweep him away.

As darkness rolled over him, he remembers hearing voices: *He's not going to make it* and *Please, God, no* echoing through his mind and tearing through his heart. In his mother's voice he heard grief and love so deep he pushed hard through the haze so he might hear it again—to know she would love him exactly as he was.

When he did, in that moment he chose life.

***

When you hear a singular narrative your whole life, it's almost impossible not to believe it. In Morgan's case, the narrative was so damaging it divided him from his family for years and nearly cost him his life.

During his adolescence, he grew increasingly worried his family would disown him, when in fact he found only support and love from them. At the time, though, Morgan would have been in the minority with his family experience.

According to a 2008-09 NTDS study, 57 percent of trans people experienced significant family rejection when they came out, which could take the form of domestic abuse, being kicked out of the house, and strained emotional bonds.[180] On the flip side, having a support system from family members has shown to be immensely beneficial in protecting trans people from the institutional obstacles threating well-being, including:

- HIV infection
- experiencing homelessness
- incarceration
- attempted suicide
- and drug and alcohol abuse.[181]

Morgan found both emotional and financial support from his family when he decided he was ready to start taking testosterone supplements in his early to mid-twenties. He was still living in his home state of North Carolina at the time, where doctors who specialized in gay health were few and far between.

He found a doctor through the trans underground network in Charlotte who prescribed him testosterone based on Morgan's informed consent. He was lucky, in that sense, because he didn't have to jump through a bunch of hoops or wait a year while a psychiatrist poked and prodded his innermost thoughts to determine whether he truly was the gender he knew himself to be. For example, though 78 percent of

---

180 Jaime M. Grant et al., *Injustice at Every Turn: A Report of the National Transgender Discrimination Survey* (Washington DC: National Center for Transgender Equality and National Gay and Lesbian Task Force, 2011), 101, accessed June 8, 2020.

181 Ibid.

respondents in the 2015 NTDS survey reported wanting to receive hormone therapy related to gender transition, only 49 percent had ever received it.[182]

The testosterone was the start of a new beginning for Morgan. His college friend had started on T supplements a couple months prior, and Morgan was excited to start to see the changes his friend was already seeing.

When his voice began to drop, Morgan was so enthused he started practicing his "Hello" every chance he got.

In front of the mirror: "Hello."

No, deeper.

Answering the phone: "Hello."

Ooh too deep.

Running to greet the knock at the door: "Hello."

Aha perfect!

"If you say 'hello' one more time, I swear..." his mom snipped.

But Morgan just grinned and resumed trying to pick up the coffee table because his newfound muscles had given him super strength which would be wasted if he didn't show it off.

---

182 James et al., *The Report of the 2015*, 99.

Before starting his physical transformation, Morgan had expected he would have to deal with a lot of backlash, that everyone would just erupt in rage or disgust around him. For the most part, though, he found acceptance from his family, friends, and coworkers, for which he considers himself fortunate.

Positive physical changes aside, however, traversing the additional social complexities which came with his new appearance brought forth fresh challenges.

Dating, in particular, proved a further ordeal. After moving out of North Carolina to DC, he felt like he could be pretty open in terms of his gender and sexuality because the laws and culture were certainly more accepting and inclusive of the LGBTQ+ community.

Nevertheless, he still grappled with the question of *When do I tell them?*

If he was out on a date with a woman, did he have the obligation to tell her he was trans right off the bat?

What if that put her off?

What if she felt like he was hiding something from her if he didn't tell her right away?

What about the very real threat of transphobia?

These internal dating struggles are something to which many in the trans community can relate. After hearing their whole life they are not "natural," it can be difficult to believe anyone would see them in a romantic or sexual way, and sometimes it feels easier to exist in the bubble where their potential partner doesn't know their whole identity.[183]

"I always start from the assumption that the possibility of a relationship is over the moment I mention I'm trans," admits Jen Richards, a trans woman actress and activist.[184]

She's not speaking theoretically; she's speaking from experience: "There was this one situation where I met a guy on an airplane. I travel a lot. We had talked for a week. I really liked him a lot. After we started emailing one day, he looked up my email address and found links to me. He emailed me an hour before our date and said, 'I just found out what you are. I have no interest in that. Goodbye.'"[185]

Reading that, some may feel sympathetic toward Jen. After all, she hadn't said or done anything to put off the guy. Being rejected solely on the basis of your identity is a hard pill to swallow.

But some may side with the guy on this one. He has every right to call off the date based on personal sexual preferences, doesn't he?

This brings up a crucial point of contention: is refusing to date trans people transphobic?

---

183 Nico Lang, "Looking for Love and Acceptance: Dating While Trans in America," Daily Beast, last modified July 12, 2017.

184 Ibid.

185 Ibid.

To answer this, let's use a logic test. The "but-for" test is a legal conception used to determine actual causation by asking, "but for the existence of X, would Y have occurred?"[186]

The "but-for" test has been used in civil rights case as an indicator of discriminatory practices. For example, Diane Schroer, a retired US Army Colonel and counterterrorism expert, was offered a job as a terrorism analyst at the Library of Congress' Congressional Research Service. The offer was later rescinded after the Library discovered Schroer was transgender. The ACLU filed a sex discrimination lawsuit on behalf of Schroer and the court ruled the Library's conduct "amounted to discrimination "because of . . . sex" under the law."[187]

Schroer v. Billington points to the fact Diane's job offer was not retracted due to the candidate's qualifications, but for the fact the candidate was transgender, pointing to clear discrimination based on transphobia.[188]

If we were to take this same logic and apply it to Jen's case, we would see initially Jen and her airplane friend had a mutual connection and hit it off. For the first week, there were no red flags. It wasn't until airplane guy found out Jen was trans that he immediately called off future interactions. But for the fact Jen is trans, airplane guy would not have stopped talking to her in that manner.

---

186 "But-for test," Cornell Law School, Legal Information Institute, accessed September 7, 2020.

187 "Schroer v. Billington," American Civil Liberties Union, accessed September 7, 2020.

188 Brynn Tannehill, "Is Refusing to Date Trans People Transphobic?" Advocate, December 14, 2019.

Is that illegal? Of course not. Is it wrong? Again, everyone has their own sexual preferences and should be allowed to decide if they don't want to date someone.

But this example does highlight the ways our society continues to operate under assumptions of cisnormativity and perpetuate cissexism.

> Cisnormativity is defined as "the expectation that all people are cissexual, that those assigned male at birth always grow up to be men and those assigned female at birth always grow up to be women."[189]

> Cissexism is the belief cisgender identities are natural and normal, while trans' identities are inferior and illegitimate.[190]

Trans individuals must navigate these social attitudes and prejudices, which fully extend to the parameters of the dating world. They face not only rejection, but cissexist sexualization from people both disgusted and fascinated with the inner workings of their sexual anatomy.[191]

---

189 Greta R. Bauer et al., ""I don't think this is theoretical; this is our lives": how erasure impacts health care for transgender people," *Journal of the Association of Nurses in AIDS Care* 20, no. 5 (September-October 2009): 356.

190 Karen L. Blair and Rhea A. Hoskin, "Transgender exclusion from the world of dating: Patterns of acceptance and rejection of hypothetical trans dating partners as a function of sexual and gender identity," *Journal of Social and Personal Relationships* 34, no. 7 (May 2018): 2075; Julia Serano, *Whipping Girl: A Transsexual Woman on Sexism and the Scapegoating of Femininity* (Seal Press, 2016), 20.

191 Blair and Hoskin, "Transgender exclusion," 13; Serano, *Whipping*, 20.

This positions trans people as a group whose sole value is attributed to whether or not a cis person deems them attractive enough or worthy enough of a romantic relationship. This damaging narrative places the feelings and comfort of the cis person above those of the trans person and centers the sexual worthiness of a trans person solely on their gender identity, rather than the person as a whole.

Similar to the sexual dichotomy the disabled community experiences, trans people are often perceived sexually merely in terms of their bodies. The fetishization of trans people, which is especially common for trans women to experience at the hands of cis men, further demeans and others them. Their bodies are often viewed as a "curiosity"—something to be played and experimented with, and then discarded when their partner decides to seek someone who is more "girlfriend" or "boyfriend" material.[192]

Being used only for your physical body when you didn't ask for such a situation never feels good, but it can be especially belittling when your body is made into a spectacle for the explicit purpose of fulfilling someone else's sexual fantasy.

Additionally, trans people often have complex relationships with their bodies, especially if they do not feel particularly in tune with the genitalia they were born with and still have. When someone then fetishizes their bodies for presenting one gender outwardly and having the genitalia of the opposite sex, they are using trans people for personal gain while

192 Eva Reign, "Trans Women and Femmes Speak Out About Being Fetishized," Them, July 21, 2018; Christin S. Milloy, "Beware the Chasers: "Admirers" Who Harass Trans People, "Slate, October 2, 2014.

disregarding how the body parts they find pleasure in may be body parts the trans person does not identify with or relate to.[193] Not to mention, their desires are based on making generalizations about all trans people having the same genitalia they were born with.

There is a difference between objectifying a trans person for their body and loving their body for the parts they love and feel comfortable with.

Herein lies the difference between what is known as a trans "chaser" versus someone who admires or is attracted to trans people:

> *The chaser prioritizes the transness over the actual person, whereas the admirer prioritizes interpersonal concerns.*[194]

The increasingly popular transgender porn scene, the fastest growing sector in porn, maintains the fetishism and desires of chasers, using derogatory terms like "t-girl," "tranny," and "ladyboy," and sexualizes the one thing many trans people hate the most about themselves.[195]

When you don't see trans men as men and trans women as women, when you don't see the human behind your physical desires, then you are part of the problem.

---

193 Reign, "Trans Women."
194 Rich Juzwiak, "Am I Fetishizing Trans Women as a Cis Guy Who Seeks Them Out for Sex?" Slate, August 21, 2019.
195 Mila Madison, "Transgender Fetishism and the Culture of Chasers," Maven, September 19, 2016.

Fetishizing trans bodies removes trans people's sexual autonomy and desires, promotes a hyper-sexualized narrative of trans people, and enforces cis entitlement over trans bodies which in turn can embolden sexual advances to the point of harassment, assault, and abuse.[196]

***

Unpacking all those layers of stereotypes made Morgan feel as if the dating scene was akin to walking on a tightrope— carefully picking his way down the line and trying not to hurt himself in the process. There was never really a dating pool of people he could safely dive into; instead, he had to gauge every individual and determine whether they would be unruffled or a threat.

In recent years, social liberalism, increased awareness and education, and greater positive media representation of trans people have sparked conversation and started to improve acceptance and understanding of the community. The subject of dating while trans still remains one of the more taboo topics, even among others in the LGBTQ+ community or allies.

A recent study on transgender exclusion in the dating realm found only 12 percent of all 958 participants would be open to dating a trans man or trans woman. Separating participants by sexual orientation:

- only 1.8 percent of straight women and 3.3 percent of straight men indicated they would date a trans person

---

196 Reign, "Trans Women."

- only 11.5 percent of gay men and 29 percent of lesbians were trans-inclusive
- bisexual/queer/non-binary participants were the group most open to dating a trans person; but even so, nearly half (48 percent) indicated they would not.[197]

That is a function of cis-generated norms and ideals for romantic partners propagated by the cis majority to the detriment of trans people. In reality, though faced with a dating scene fraught with obstacles and hazards, healthy relationships still prevail.

***

Morgan, once he got a knack for reading his romantic interests, had plenty of "normal," healthy relationships with "normal," healthy ups and downs like any relationship. They ended not because of anything to do with his being trans, but just as a product of two incompatible people.

He tells the story of one woman he dated who he met at a gym and on their first date they went to a bar for drinks. He had never told a date he was trans before, and he wasn't sure how to proceed. He decided the best way forward was to just get to know her, like on any first date.

As someone who grew up in a household full of storytelling, and a storyteller and writer himself, Morgan loved words. They were his upbringing and his anchor and his awakening. So, he turned to his date and asked her the big question:

---

197 Blair and Hoskin, "Transgender exclusion," 7.

"What are your favorite books?"

She paused, and Morgan says he got excited, thinking: *Such an avid reader, she has to weigh and sift all the genres and titles and authors swimming through her head.*

Finally, she snorted, "My favorite books? Silly—I don't read."

For a man of many words, that response left Morgan speechless.

Oh god, he thought, *who did I agree to go out with?* With nothing else to say and nothing left to lose, he thought, *Fuck it.*

"Well, I'm trans."[198]

The story of "Bookless," as Morgan's friends so affectionately call her, is a funny one and a crowd pleaser, but the point Morgan highlights is relationships involving trans people are not hinged upon a person being trans. After Morgan revealed his identity to his date (and then explained what being a trans man meant), she really had no issue with his gender identity.

It was Morgan who ultimately ended the relationship, as date after date they just didn't click. Because who doesn't like books?

When he tells this story, he adds if he ever ran into "Bookless" again, he would thank her, "because if it weren't for

---

198 *Story District*, "Morgan Givens in Story District's Top Shelf," February 4, 2016, video, 10:16.

her, I would still believe my relationships would end or fail to begin because of the physicality of my body, and that just isn't true."[199]

Though it may seem so at first, Morgan's dating life, his gender identity journey, and his continuing sexual health battles are not all tied up in one dominant narrative. He feared for much of his adolescence the sting of rejection, abuse, even death; but what he eventually found was acceptance, love, and a truer life with his mom, his brother, his grandmother, his friends, and his wife.

To say the themes of his story ring true for most or even many other trans people, or to say Morgan does not and will not continue to confront immense hurdles on his walk of life, would sadly be wholly untrue. Yet his story and the stories of countless other trans people in the US who have fought and continue to fight hard to get where they are today are reflective of the tremendous resilience of transgender people as one of the most marginalized communities in this country.

The challenges trans individuals confront are a function of systemic discrimination against the community, translating to a lack of legal protection, violence, stigma, harassment, lack of access to education and employment, and lack of health care coverage.[200] It falls upon the shoulders of the rest of us to continue disrupting the negative stereotypes and stigmas surrounding the trans community, to dispel the notions of objectification and hyper-sexualization, and

---

199 Ibid.
200 "Understanding the Transgender Community," Human Rights Campaign, accessed October 6, 2020.

to understand the specific struggles they deal with every day. It is our responsibility as collective supporters to carry these conversations into the medical field to combat discrimination and mistreatment and break down the structures that uphold transphobia.

Above all, it begins with recognizing trans is human.

CHAPTER 11

More Than a Pinch

Bursts of laughter and snippets of excited chatter roll through the house, bouncing across busy hands, curling over hooks, ducking through precise loops of yarn, and dancing across a quick smile as their lips draw upward. Calls of *"Chalo chalo, time thai gayo"* (let's go, it's time) ring through the town center as more bodies fill the space, eager to begin their works of art. And the pieces they create surely are just that, taking the form perhaps of a "'pretty-in-pink doll', or a cuddly sheep, or a flamboyant wall hanging."[201]

The women gathered at the Happy Threads meeting are members of the Dawoodi Bohras, a Shiite branch of Islam, which is primarily based in Gujarat, India but has pockets with members all over the globe.[202]

Many of the women will design and create ridas at the gatherings, the traditional form of dress for Bohra women unlike any other garment found in the Muslim world. The two-piece dress consists of a long skirt which flows from the waist to the ankles, and a shawl-like top covering the chest, arms, and

---

201 Mariya Zoeb, "Happy Threads— Know Our World," The Dawoodi Bohras, November 8, 2019.

202 "The Bohras Today," The Dawoodi Bohras, accessed March 27, 2020.

head with an opening for the face. Elaborate embroidery, lace, or crochet work adorns every piece atop a striking medley of colorful, patterned fabric. The end result is a garment-quickly-turned-fashion-icon which blends traditionalist Islamic requirements that call for the coverage and limited exposure of a woman's figure with the functionality and aesthetic preferred by modern Bohra women.[203]

This idea of blending age-old traditions with modern values is crucial to how the Dawoodi Bohras follow their faith and conduct their lives today.

Above all, the Bohra's value system is grounded in love and the fostering of good will. Their teachings and faith exude peacefulness, mindfulness, and the avoidance of conflict by seeking common ground. Community building is at the core of their principles, as they strive to understand and facilitate dialogue with different communities, sects, and religions around the world, and continually explore how their community can progress themselves and better the world around them.[204]

Whether through providing the latest in medical care, ensuring quality education and professional opportunities for both boys and girls, empowering the less fortunate, or launching environmental protection initiatives, this Muslim community of just under one million promotes a broader social impact than its relatively small numbers may otherwise suggest.

---

203 "Attire & Tradition," The Dawoodi Bohras, accessed March 27, 2020.
204 "The Da`I Al-Mutlaq," The Dawoodi Bohras, accessed March 27, 2020.

Their social impact extends around the globe as communities of Bohras have and continue to migrate and settle in search of better prospects or a new life.[205] In the US, there are many thriving Bohra communities—in San Francisco, Houston, Chicago, and Philadelphia. Just across the Delaware River from Philly, you'll find them in bustling Camden, New Jersey, too.

Camden was home to Tasneem Raja, an Indian-American girl born to Indian and Pakistani immigrants in the early 80s. Raised in one of many US-Bohra communities, or as she refers to it, "[a] controversial, secretive South Asian Muslim sect," Tasneem experienced what it was like to grow up as a first-generation immigrant during a time when the standard was still white, middle-class American.[206]

Her life was a balancing act. It consisted of jeans and t-shirts, school, and trips to the mall, while also consisting of ridas, *madrassa* (religious school), and social gatherings with all the aunties and uncles. This duality of cultures is something many first—or second—generation children of immigrants simultaneously grapple with and celebrate.[207]

Tasneem's upbringing, however, left her with lifelong trauma and forced her to question some of her faith's values.

---

205 "The Bohras Today," The Dawoodi Bohras.

206 Tasneem Raja, "I Underwent Genital Mutilation as a Child—Right Here in the United States," *Mother Jones*, April 21, 2017.

207 Mariya Taher, "The Duality of My Life: Growing Up a Hybrid of American and Dawoodi Bohra," *Brown Girl Magazine*, January 10, 2018.

***

At the tender age of seven, her mother brought Tasneem to the house of a family acquaintance one brisk morning. Gripping Tasneem's hand, her mother ushered her up the walkway and through the front door into an unassuming foyer.

Inside, it was quiet, cold, and dim. The mood hung somber and low over their heads. Tasneem could feel the beat of her mother's heart through the palm of her hand, pressed squarely now against Tasneem's back. She nudged Tasneem forward as two unfamiliar Indian aunties appeared from down a long hallway. Her mother's hand lifted from her back in a final push forward, and Tasneem felt the absence of her touch like slap to the face.

Faltering, she turned questioning eyes onto her mother's face before one of the aunties clasped her arm and guided her down the dark hallway. They brought Tasneem into a bedroom and forcibly held her down on a mattress. As she frantically squirmed and wriggled to free herself, they wrenched her underwear down and a glint of silver scissors flashed before her eyes.

Just like the ones my dad uses to trim his beard she thought, before the blades disappeared between her legs.[208]

Tasneem describes it as a "tight, mean little pinch" between her legs, but the reality is much more sickening.[209] Female genital mutilation (FGM), also known as female genital

---

circumcision or cutting, is a serious public health concern practiced worldwide.

> *FGM involves the partial or total removal of the external female genitalia for non-medical reasons. According to the World Health Organization and the United Nations Population Fund, there are no health benefits or medical justifications for FGM, and the procedure can never be safe or without risks.*[210]

The verdict is still out on exactly why FGM is performed, but the practice serves to "perpetuate discriminatory views about the status and role of women in society."[211]

- A vast majority from the Bohra and other FGM-practicing communities cite the need to inhibit a girl or woman's sexual promiscuity as the rationale, and it's often believed to be a rite of passage for girls transitioning into womanhood.[212]
- In many FGM-practicing communities, women who do not have the procedure done are seen as dirty, impure, and of lower status, and are often considered unmarriageable.[213]

---

210 "Female genital mutilation," World Health Organization, last modified February 3, 2020; "Female genital mutilation," United Nations Population Fund, accessed March 27, 2020.

211 Archana Pyati and Claudia De Palma, *Female Genital Mutilation: Protecting Girls and Women in the U.S. from FGM and Vacation Cutting* (New York: Sanctuary for Families, 2013), 5.

212 Pyati and De Palma, *Female Genital*, 5; "What is Female Genital Mutilation?" Amnesty International, accessed March 27, 2020, 3.

213 Pyati and De Palma, *Female Genital*, 5, 6; "What is Female," Amnesty International, 3; World Health Organization, *Eliminating female genital mutilation: an interagency statement* (Geneva, Switzerland: WHO, 2008), 6.

- In the US, immigrant parents and relatives who choose to continue the practice on their daughters may desire to maintain their child's identity with the culture of their country of origin, and they may see it as a way to protect their daughters from Western influence while reinforcing their traditional customs.[214]

FGM can range in severity from the partial removal of the clitoris (type 1) to the cutting and narrowing of the vaginal opening (type 3, also known as infibulation).[215] In the Bohra community, the decision is left up to the discretion of whoever is holding the knife.

Though most often the more severe or invasive procedures are associated with greater health risks, all forms of FGM provoke harm to the victim.

Immediate complications can include:

- severe pain
- acute painful urination
- shock
- fever
- excessive bleeding
- infections
- injury and/or swelling of genital tissue
- and death.

---

214 Pyati and De Palma, *Female Genital*, 7; Michael Miller and Francesca Moneti, *Changing a Harmful Social Convention: Female Genital Mutilation/Cutting* (Florence, Italy: UNICEF, 2008), 11. Accessed March 27, 2020.

215 "Female genital mutilation," World Health Organization.

Long-term complications can include:

- prolonged urinary issues
- vaginal problems (discharge, itching, bacterial vaginosis and other infections)
- painful and difficult menstruation
- scar tissue
- unendurable pain during intercourse and decreased satisfaction
- increased risk of childbirth complications (prolonged and difficult labor, excessive bleeding, etc.) and newborn deaths
- need for later reconstructive surgeries
- and lasting psychological trauma.[216]

So, although the shock, pain, and trauma of the violation may have warranted Tasneem to reduce that moment in her mind to a pinch, the reality of the situation was much more severe, and that day continued to haunt her.

***

Locked away for purposes of self-preservation, the memory resurfaced years later when Tasneem was thirteen. It was her freshman year, and her teacher was showing a video of a young African girl being prepared for her ritual mutilation by village elders, much the same as Tasneem had been forced down on a mattress by the two aunties.

The imagery tickled a memory of a recurring dream she had for years following the incident in which, "the lower half of

---

216 Ibid.

my body was made of kid's construction toys, and pieces kept breaking off as I frantically tried to keep myself together."[217]

At lunch later, she recalls her white girlfriends expressing relief over the fact they didn't have to worry about FGM happening here in America.

Feelings of shame and confusion slithered their way into the back of Tasneem's mind. She recalls later how, due to the extreme secrecy surrounding the practice, there was this feeling among her and her friends of, *"Did that really happen?"* FGM is so hush-hush within the Bohra community many girls don't even realize it is a common practice until later, and many of the men have no knowledge of it at all.

"For the longest time, I didn't even know other people had this done, too," one friend revealed to Tasneem. "I thought it was something my mom only did to me, and I didn't know why."[218]

But the unfortunate truth is FGM is a reality for thousands of American women, and a threat for generations of girls to come.

***

In 2012, the Center for Disease Control and Prevention revealed more than half a million women and girls were affected by, or at risk of, FGM in the United States. These

---

217 Raja, "I Underwent."
218 Ibid.

numbers are extrapolated by applying country-and age-specific FGM/C prevalence rates to the number of US women and girls with connections to those countries.[219] Each year, girls and women are subjected to illegal cutting on US soil by traditional practitioners or health care providers who support or don't question the practice of FGM. Families may also send their daughters abroad to undergo the procedure, a process known as "vacation cutting."[220]

The number of girls at risk doesn't seem to be waning, even as the US appears to be moving toward a more sexually liberated and progressive society for females. In fact, the number of women and girls who are victims of, or at risk for mutilation tripled from 1990 to 2012.[221]

These numbers can partially be explained by the rapid increase in the number of immigrants entering the US from countries with a high prevalence of FGM over the past several decades.[222]

By the early 1960s, change was beginning to ripple across the US as the civil rights movement gathered momentum and followers to its cause. Changing attitudes helped to push forward immigration reform which abolished an antiquated

---

219 Mark Mather and Charlotte Feldman-Jacobs, "Women and Girls at Risk of Female Genital Mutilation/Cutting in the United States," Population Reference Bureau, February 5, 2016.

220 Pyati and De Palma, Female Genital, ii.

221 Howard Goldberg et al., "Female Genital Mutilation/Cutting in the United States: Updated Estimates of Women and Girls at Risk, 2012," Public Health Reports 131, no. 2 (March-April 2016): 340.

222 Mather and Feldman-Jacobs, "Women and Girls."

national origins quota system grounded in discriminatory principles.[223]

The Immigration and Naturalization Act of 1965 created a new policy intent on reuniting immigrant families and building a skilled labor force from abroad in the US. The demographic effects were almost immediate. Immigration from Asian countries, especially Southeast Asia, more than quadrupled over the next five years, and by the 1990s people of Asian descent comprised 31 percent of the immigrant population, up from only 6 percent in the 1950s.[224]

Families like Tasneem's uprooted their lives at the promise of the American dream, bringing with them their cultures and customs. For some, this meant the ritual cutting or mutilation, or as Bohras call it *khatna*, of their daughters as well.

***

In Tasneem's case, she recalls in her teens and twenties almost naively believing the practice would peter out in the Bohra community as families assimilated and the first generation of Bohras born in America began their own families. That hope was crushed, though, as she witnessed women her age or younger continuing to arrange *khatna* for their own daughters.

Tasneem attributes, in large part, the tight control the Bohra community has over its members and the severe consequences dissidents face to FGM remaining unchecked.

---

223 "U.S. Immigration Since 1965," History, last modified June 7, 2019.
224 Ibid.

As she points out, "Bohras feel tremendous pressure to conform. There's this fear of angering the clergy. And so, you might think some women would just lie, you know, and say their daughters had this done when they didn't. But Bohras believe that their leaders are all-seeing and so...they're afraid to do that. A Bohra woman talking to a reporter last week said this is like a cult. You know, it feels like we have a tyrant over us and there's this whole control thing going on."[225]

So, they pray in private for the practice to end, secretly weep when their daughters are born, and stay silent.

Tasneem understands the drastic consequences of speaking out against Bohra customs all too well. When she tried to bring up *khatna* to her parents, in particular her mother, she made little headway in having a productive conversation or reversing their opinions.

She argues, "as in many rigid orthodoxies, the burden of social policing in the Bohra community falls largely on women, who have the most to lose from rocking the boat and who are often suffering from unacknowledged personal trauma of their own."[226]

Members exhibiting rebellious tendencies can face excommunication and social boycott, with negative effects rippling out to impact family members as well. Rather than work toward a common ground of understanding,

225 Tasneem Raja, interview by Ari Shapiro and Audie Cornish, *All Things Considered*, NPR, April 24, 2017.
226 Raja, "I Underwent."

Tasneem and her parents became polarized forces estranged from one another.[227]

***

Tasneem's procedure removed a pinch of skin from the clitoral hood and left emotional burdens, but no lasting physical trauma.[228] For many FGM survivors, though, physical consequences can follow them throughout their adult lives.

Mariya Karimjee, another member of the Dawoodi Bohras, was also seven when she had, as her mother called it, her "bug" cut. When she was fifteen, armed with the book *Our Bodies, Ourselves*, some internet research, and rumblings of betrayal, she confronted her mother.[229]

Her mother's explanation was clumsy, something about cutting her clitoris because women shouldn't be sexual.

"You removed the part of me that makes me feel good while having sex?" Mariya asked.[230]

She says at that moment, "I thought I knew. I thought I appreciated exactly what had been taken away from me."[231]

---

227 Ibid.
228 Ibid.
229 Mariya Karimjee, "Who Do We Think We Are?" *This American Life*, May 6, 2016.
230 Ibid.
231 Ibid.

But Mariya's procedure not only shortened her clitoris—it had also left her with extensive scar tissue and nerve damage.[232] She wasn't just missing the part of her which might make sex more enjoyable. Mariya's cut had set her up for a life of painful sex.

In college, when she first began experimenting with masturbation, she quickly discovered achieving an orgasm was not going to come easily. One wrong move and her entire body was laced through with pain.

But she didn't tell anyone. Inundated in the infamous hookup culture, she put on a façade even around friends who were privy to her secret. "I would pretend I was just like them. I'd assure them I was hooking up randomly with people, same as they were. It's ridiculous, I know, but I didn't know what to do."[233]

The doctors she visited largely seemed at a loss with what to do with her as well. Her first gynecological checkup was performed by a doctor who tried to make Maryia as comfortable as possible, but who was not well-versed on clitorectomies and couldn't do much herself to help. Over the following years, Mariya received a lot of winces and grimaces at the sight between her legs. At lot of over-apologetic explanations and condescending pats and sympathetic "oh dears."

When she began dating, she waited months before she told her boyfriend why she kept rejecting his advances

---

232 Ibid.
233 Ibid.

past second base. At the year mark, she finally decided she needed to just do it; she could just push through the pain of sex. Mariya told her boyfriend to keep going no matter what, chugged half a bottle of wine to calm her nerves, and guided him to the bed.

But as soon as they started, Mariya recalls, "Pain shot up my body. I could feel it in my teeth and in the muscles of my jaw. My insides felt like they were being sandpapered. The pain was everywhere."[234]

As she sat in the bed afterwards, crying, Mariya wondered if she would ever want to try having sex again, a thought which terrified her.

"It wasn't just that I was scared of sex," she admits, "but that because of that, true love would escape me forever, that I was unlovable."[235]

Confused, angry, and seeking answers, she finally turned to her mom. Pouring out her fears and burdens, Mariya connected with her mom that night over the phone in a way she never had before.

Her mom revealed she too would experience pain sometimes during sex, but through conversation and experimentation, she and her husband had figured out a way to make it work. She said she had sexual desires too, and just wanted to feel like the women in the Harlequin romances.

---

234 Ibid.
235 Ibid.

"I hate everyone else too," her mom let out just before they hung up, "Those women on TV who love sex, who enjoy it, I hate them too."[236]

It's a sentiment to which many facing any type of sexual dysfunction or sexual pain may relate. Casual, easy-breezy sex, often painted as a universal reality in popular culture and media, is not the case for many people. FGM is also such a difficult form of sexual dysfunction because it is born from violence underpinned by cultural and familial ties and values.

FGM is often performed when the victims are too young to entirely comprehend what's happening and the trauma might not resurface until years later, as with both Tasneem and Mariya. That can bring feelings of confusion and betrayal toward your loved ones, and a questioning of your identity as the implications are fully digested.

As Fatoumata Jatta, an FGM survivor from a large, loving Gambian family, notes from her experience:

"My story of being cut, surviving the practice, and living with the consequences has often felt so removed from my understanding of my own identity, and I've had to learn to integrate this part of me so that I can accept myself fully. Intellectually I have always understood that if my grandmother had me cut as a baby, it was because she absolutely thought it was the best thing for me, that for her it was the right thing to do. But emotionally I've had to understand and make sense

---

236 Ibid.

of the feelings I was left with: confusion, anger, shame, powerlessness, loss, and grief."[237]

Or Maryia Taher, who was cut at the age of seven during a vacation to India:

"I honestly had a great childhood, so it's really hard for me to talk about this [FGM]. I feel that people paint me as the picture of a victim, and I hate that. Yes, that was a violent thing that was done to me, but it's also such a complicated form of violence."[238]

Complicating the matter further, the act *and* the implications behind FGM—that women should not have sexual desires—entangle the violence and sexually repressive morals with survivors' sense of sexuality. Some survivors internalize those messages and feel guilty for desiring sex or feel as if they are unworthy of sexual contentment.[239] Others, like Fatoumata, struggle with feeling as if an integral piece of their womanhood is gone, irrevocably altered, or violated.

"For me it has been a process of accepting many things," Fatoumata reflects, "that being cut doesn't make me any more of a woman, as my grandmother believed, but neither does it make me any less of one, as I believed."[240]

---

237 Matthew Tucker, "These British Women Are All Survivors Of Female Genital Mutilation," Buzzfeed News, July 16, 2016.

238 Sonia Moghe, "3 US women share the horrors of female genital mutilation," CNN, May 11, 2017.

239 Maria Lobo, "Consider the potential emotional and psychological consequences of female genital mutilation" (Senior Thesis, Imperial College London), accessed October 6, 2020, 6.

240 Tucker, "These British Women."

***

The sad truth is it does not appear as if the practice of FGM in the US is dying out or will die out naturally. Every so often, a story about girls being cut in America will surface: the culprits are presented, the survivors share their stories, the general public is horrified, and then the story is forgotten. It creates this sense of hopelessness for Tasneem and her Bohra friends because every time a woman comes forward, the community simply pretends it's not happening or places the blame somewhere else.[241]

In April 2017, an Indian-American doctor was arrested in Michigan which made the issue of FGM within the Bohra community a lot harder to ignore.

The forty-four-year-old emergency room physician, Jumana Nagarwala, along with two other followers of the Bohra sect, were charged with performing FGM on two seven-year-old girls from Bohra families, one of whom "could barely walk afterward."[242] This was the first case of its kind in the United States, which is baffling since FGM has been illegal in the US for over twenty years.

There is hope this case could raise awareness and spur a larger movement. Tasneem admits the arrest and national attention could pressure the clergy and inspire more survivors within the Bohra community to speak out.

---

241 Tasneem Raja, interview by Ari Shapiro and Audie Cornish, *All Things Considered*, NPR.

242 Jacey Fortin, "Michigan Doctor Is Accused of Genital Cutting of 2 Girls," *The New York Times*, April 13, 2017.

But she also fears backlash from the public, especially during these times of growing Islamophobia. She echoes sentiments of others in her community who worry everyday Bohras will be targeted for crimes for which the leadership is responsible.

"The only way this practice will end," Tasneem argues, "is if the clergy unequivocally comes out and tells Bohras it's time to stop and… offers support to women and girls who have already experienced it."[243]

The case of Jumana Nagarwala brought national attention to the issue and to the practices of the Dawoodi Bohra community. But just as Tasneem mentions, it would be naive to believe all, or even the majority of, Bohras believe in or participate in FGM practices, or that they are the only community within the US which subjects its girls and women to this ritual.

In fact, it is estimated 97 percent of women and girls at risk for FGM in the US are from African countries, while only 3 percent are from Asian countries.[244] Additionally, this custom predates religion and has no religious grounding in either Christianity or Islam, though communities and members of both faiths continue the practice to "purify" their daughters.[245]

In 2016, Renee Bergstrom, a white woman from a midwestern Christian family, came forward with her story. She was

243 Tasneem Raja, interview by Ari Shapiro and Audie Cornish, *All Things Considered*, NPR.

244 Mather and Feldman-Jacobs, "Women and Girls."

245 Lucy Wescott, "Female Genital Mutilation on the Rise in the U.S.," Newsweek, February 6, 2015.

cut when she was three years old after her mother saw her masturbating. She took Renee to a church clinic where they performed FGM on girls who masturbated. At fifteen, Renee unwittingly went back to the same clinic to ask about a tugging sensation caused by her scar tissue and was shamed by the doctor about the sin of self-pleasuring.[246]

She says she wanted to start speaking out about her experience because of "concern regarding increased hatred and disrespect toward women, other cultures, and religions—as if Christians in the United States had a flawless history. FGM is not my shame, it is my story. I witnessed Christian religions declaring masturbation a sin, 'some Christian leaders and doctors' recommending circumcision to prevent it, physicians carrying out the practice and our American culture first accepting this form of sexual abuse and then denying it ever occurred."[247]

FGM is not a practice solely relegated to non-Western cultures and is a violation overlooked by and perpetuated within American society. Yet, the US has been slow to develop an effective legal framework to protect those at risk of FGM. The practice was made explicitly illegal in the US in 1996, but, "legislation criminalizing the practice has not been comprehensively implemented or enforced, and community members, social service providers and law enforcement officials often fail to identify, report or investigate incidents of FGM."[248]

---

246 Renee Bergstrom, "FGM happened to me in white, midwest America," The Guardian, December 3, 2016; Moghe, "3 US women."
247 Bergstrom, "FGM happened."
248 Pyati and De Palma, *Female Genital*, iii.

The same year FGM was criminalized, money was appropriated for the Department of Health and Human Services to conduct a study on FGM prevalence in the US, as well as to implement outreach and educational activities in FGM-practicing communities, yet none of these activities have been realized. In 2013, long after many other countries had passed similar protections, the US finally criminalized the process of "vacation cutting" when President Obama signed the Transport for Female Genital Mutilation Act. Unfortunately, the practice of sending girls abroad under the ruse of a summer vacation trip remains prevalent today.[249]

The passage of such laws sends a clear message the United States condemns FGM as a criminal act with serious consequences, but as noted with the Nagarwala case, an enforcement gap continues to exist with FGM legislation. The Nagarwala case was the first federal FGM prosecution and only one criminal FGM case has been prosecuted under a state statute.[250]

There are several reasons why the enforcement gap exists:

- FGM is a gendered issue and a result of deep-rooted inequality between the sexes. Therefore, it is an issue

---

249 Pyati and De Palma, *Female Genital*, iii; "Vacation Cutting: An Illegal Practice Still Running Rampant," AHA Foundation, accessed June 18, 2020.

250 Pyati and De Palma, *Female Genital*, 14; Annie McCallum, "LaGrange crime: Woman charged with female genital mutilation, 2nd-degree cruelty to children," *Ledger-Enquirer*, last modified March 11, 2010; Julia Lalla-Maharajh, "Female Genital Mutilation in Georgia, USA," HuffPost, last modified December 6, 2017.

which, like many female human rights issues, is neglected and ignored.[251]

- Oftentimes, "women and girls who have been subject to FGM frequently feel too disempowered, are too young, or remain silent about their traumatic experience to speak up and raise the number of prosecutions."[252]

- A lack of laws at the state or local level specifically banning FGM, which is the case for twenty-four states, make it more difficult to report on or prosecute FGM cases.[253]

- Child abuse statutes in many states allow for cultural exceptions when it comes to medical decisions, confusing legal responsibility to inform authorities over suspected or actual cases of FGM.[254]

  - Within the medical field, though FGM performed on US soil is generally performed by traditional practitioners hailing from countries where the practice is commonplace, some US health care providers may also perform FGM because they do not want to question the patient's cultural beliefs and practices.[255]

  - The American Academy of Pediatrics (AAP) even briefly endorsed so-called "symbolic" FGM procedures involving "clitoral nicks," or small cuts made under the clitoral hood under local anesthesia, to appease patients' "perceived cultural requirements" without performing more extensive injury.[256]

---

251 Soraya Kamali-Nafar, "Why FGM in the US is Rarely Prosecuted," Women In International Security, July 13, 2018.

252 Ibid.

253 Pyati and De Palma, *Female Genital*, 14.

254 Ibid.

255 Pyati and De Palma, *Female Genital*, 10.

256 Ibid.

Silence around this issue is one of the root causes as to why laws criminalizing FGM in the US are still so ineffective. It leaves many girls vulnerable, girls who don't even know this is happening to others in their community or in the US, and who don't know how to speak up against it. The secrecy fuels shame, which continues the tradition of silence.

The general lack of awareness about FGM within our borders on the part of the American public additionally creates a system which allows the practice to persist behind closed doors or on school vacations.

Amanda Parker, the senior director of the AHA Foundation says, "Every time I talk to people about the work we do with regards to FGM, the response is always shock: 'That happens here (in the US)?' I think we are up against a big learning curve."[257]

Educators who are working directly with at-risk girls and their communities need appropriate training on FGM and on the deeply entrenched cultural beliefs and customs which underlie and perpetuate the practice. Informing about warning signs or how to best approach families and communities is critical to ensuring laws are enforced, and vulnerable girls are better protected.[258]

In addition, having conversations with young girls outside of the influence of their families and communities about the dangers of FGM can arm them with information and

---

257 "Vacation Cutting," AHA Foundation.
258 Ibid.

empower them to resist their family's wishes. Many girls who are old enough to understand the implications of the procedure still do not resist their family simply because they have no knowledge of the ritual and believe it will be the best thing for them.[259]

Health care providers also need training on the medical consequences of FGM and, depending on the type and severity of an individual case, an understanding of how to adapt their practices to accommodate survivors' needs. There are doctors in the US who specialize in survivors of FGM, both gynecologists and plastic surgeons, who work to reverse the procedure and restore sensation to the clitoris.

Mariya Karimjee, after another failed sexual encounter, found such a specialist who had examined other women and girls who had been cut. Unlike her previous doctors, this one was able to give Mariya a comprehensive explanation of her anatomy, scarring, and what it would mean for her sex life.[260] Because FGM specialists are so far and few between, many gynecologists confronted with an FGM patient for the first time may not know where to turn for information and guidance, or where to refer their patient.[261] More education and better data on the prevalence of this issue in Western countries can help to increase awareness and improve medical inclusivity.

For example, at Heartlands Hospital in Birmingham, UK, data reporting treatment of 1,500 cases of FGM over the past

---

259 Pyati and De Palma, *Female Genital*, 8.

260 Karimjee, "Who Do We."

261 Aryn Baker, "Doctors Around the World Rally for New Surgery to Counter Female Genital Mutilation," *Time*, March 21, 2017.

five years has led to the recognition that survivors of FGM have specific health care needs, such as psychological trauma and the need for increased attention during childbirth due to pain.[262]

We have a tendency in the US, when we hear about female genital mutilation, to think of it as something which happens thousands of miles away across the ocean in a mud hut with a dirty knife. But FGM is an *international* issue, and it would be irresponsible to think of it as some distant horror.

Furthermore, it would be irresponsible not to include FGM as a topic of discussion in conversations about sexual health concerns, in favor of leaving the practice and survivors in the dark, dusty corner so as not to tarnish the spotless facade of American liberty. Just like all of the issues discussed in this book, if we aren't having the uncomfortable conversations and bringing awareness to overlooked sexual health problems, we cannot move toward sexual liberation. As is blatantly clear with this human rights violation, freedom of sexual health and sexuality is critical to overall individual freedom.

---

262 Wescott, "Female Genital."

PART 3

DISCOVERING VENUS

CHAPTER 12

Brick by Brick

Throughout this book, we've taken an in-depth look at some of the issues and people commonly left out of the sex positivity and sexual health sphere. The stories explored the intersection of sexuality and sexual dysfunction, menstrual health, and societal stigmas. But the key to understanding why we need better female sexual health care and awareness is recognizing the intersections within the intersections.

These issues and these people do not exist within a vacuum. The lack of attention paid to female sexual health is not just an issue of inequality between the sexes which dismisses the validity of female sexuality and threatens the integrity of female bodies. It is also an issue of racism, ableism, classism, and discrimination against the LGBTQ+ community. The more layered the systemic inequalities, the more vulnerable the individual.

***

Laura Kiesel, a journalist and blogger who often reports on her own personal experiences at the intersection of chronic illness, sexual health, and socioeconomic status, is someone who is familiar with facing multiple barriers to appropriate health care. She has suffered from endometriosis for most of her life, first experiencing extremely painful periods which were most likely a result of her condition around age twelve. Laura came across the term "endometriosis" a few years later, but her family was in no position financially to afford the laparoscopic surgery necessary to confirm a diagnosis and to treat the condition.

With no way to properly treat or confirm her condition, Laura just had to live with the heavy bleeding and intense cramps knocking her out every month.

Then, around the age of nineteen, she began to experience severe gastrointestinal distress. Everything she ate seemed to go right through her. She lost twenty pounds in one semester and had to take a medical leave of absence. But when she went to see her doctors about it, they dismissed her because she "looked healthy."

When she brought up her worsening symptoms to the college nurse and nutritionist, they told her she just needed to pursue a healthier diet and to stop being so neurotic.[263] Laura refused to believe the same diet which didn't seem to affect her friends at all was making her so sick that she couldn't get out of bed. She insisted to the nurse there was something wrong with her internally:

"I'm sure there's something else going on," she pressed. "I'm pretty sure I have this thing called endometriosis. I've read it

263 Laura Kiesel, "The Burden of Invisible Illness," Medium, December 16, 2018.

can spread to all the pelvic area organs. Is it possible it could be infiltrating my intestines and causing these symptoms?"

To which the response was, "Honey, you couldn't possibly be so sick with such shiny, thick hair!"[264]

Even GI specialist doctors outright dismissed endometriosis as a contributing factor to Laura's intestinal problems, becoming condescending when she brought up a condition outside of their expertise.

She says, "I had been so often dismissed when I brought it up to other medical professionals over the years, I almost began to believe they were playing a game of reverse psychology with me—as if their egos existed to be contrarian to their patients, especially those who dared to diagnose themselves."[265]

It wasn't until she was twenty-three when she finally had the insurance coverage to offset the cost of laparoscopic surgery, during which the existence of her widespread endometriosis spreading to and strangling parts of her colon and intestines was confirmed. After her surgery, she says her GI symptoms noticeably improved by 80-90 percent after six months, and her periods, while still painful, were nothing like the horror story she endured every month before.

But, as no cure currently exists for endometriosis, in many women it will grow back, and symptoms will worsen again overtime. It's not uncommon for Laura to hear stories from

---

264 Ibid.
265 Laura Kiesel, "My First Lap— Part 1," Endometriosis.net, July 23, 2018.

other sufferers who have had half a dozen to a dozen surgeries due to recurring symptoms.

Laura's symptoms returned full force about a decade after her first surgery. She points to how this is particularly an issue because it contributes to her disabling chronic pain, an area in which not many doctors specialize. According to a 2012 study by the National Pain Report of 117 US and Canadian medical schools, less than 4 percent had a required course in pain and only one in six offered an elective class specifically on the topic of pain.[266]

As a result, there is a wide disparity among doctors in understanding pain, and specifically understanding acute versus chronic pain.

"When doctors don't even have a basic understanding of chronic pain and its anatomical and neurological effects on the body and mind, they likely also can't comprehend why and how it's disabling," Laura argues.[267]

Moreover, as Laura presents physically healthy—i.e., she doesn't have a clearly visible disability, and as a middle-aged woman is not someone we tend to associate with disability—she faces unique obstacles in getting doctors to fully comprehend her bodily state.

She encountered similar accusations of fabrication when trying to get a diagnosis of Ehlers-Danlos syndrome (EDS)—a

---

266 Elizabeth Magill, "Medical Schools Failing at Pain Education," National Pain Report, April 16, 2012.

267 Kiesel, "The Burden."

connective tissue disorder—as she did with her endome-triosis and GI symptoms. Though several doctors and physical therapists mentioned hyper-mobility as a possible explanation for Laura's pain problems during her twenties, she still did not receive a concrete EDS diagnosis until she came across the term on her own well into her thirties. After learning about EDS, it took only a few more months to get a diagnosis from a specialist.

Yet, the responsibility fell to Laura to research her own symp-toms and find possible answers and solutions. If Laura was in pain and seeking treatment for so many years, why did it take so long for her specialists to confirm her underly-ing condition?

The gap in treatment and diagnosis meant Laura had to con-stantly fight to have her illnesses taken seriously.[268]

Laura's chronic pain makes it difficult, if not impossible, to hold a full-time job. Yet, despite written documentation from doctors spelling out her accommodation needs, Laura strug-gled to secure rental modifications mandated under the Fair Housing Act, or to obtain disability status under Medicaid until she received her EDS diagnosis.[269]

Disability bias in the insurance industry is not limited to Laura's experience. A recent study reported by the Stanford Institute for Economic Policy Research found, "women fac-ing permanent or severe work-limiting impairments are 20

268 Ibid.
269 Ibid.

percent more likely than men to have their claims wrongly rejected."[270]

According to Stanford economist Luigi Pistaferri, this puts people waiting for disability insurance at a greater risk for worsening health and death. He also argues the nature of the benefits application process itself may be a contributing factor to the gender bias. At the end of the screening process, you have to list out your daily activities, answering questions like:

- Do you take care of pets?
- Do you take care of a parent?
- Do you take care of the shopping for the household?

"We think that because of the role that society has assigned to women, women are more likely than a man to say, 'I'm not sitting on the couch all day, and despite the disability, I still do the shopping and take care of the kids and my mom, etc.,'" Pistaferri says.[271]

Another study points to disability bias in age, finding younger adults were less likely to be granted disability insurance than older adults.[272] So, not only do we have this rhetoric floating around that Medicaid recipients, even those with disabling

270 May Wong, "Q&A: What's behind the gender gap in disability benefits?" Stanford Institute for Economic Policy Research (SIEPR), April 1, 2020.

271 Ibid.

272 Kalman Rupp, "Factors Affecting Initial Disability Allowance Rates for the Disability Insurance and Supplemental Security Income Programs: The Role of the Demographic and Diagnostic Composition of Applicants and Local Labor Market Conditions," *Social Security Bulletin* 72, no. 4 (November 2012): 32.

health issues, just need to work harder and stop asking for handouts, we also are making it more difficult for specific groups of people within the disabled community to access benefits based on wrongful assumptions about what disability looks like.

Couple disability prejudice with economic barriers and layer that on top of medical ignorance of female sexual health issues and implicit gender biases which devalue female pain, and you end up with a system that's against you at every turn.

And Laura is white. If we take any of these issues and put them in the context of the experiences of a racial minority, we get another picture.

***

Implicit biases in the medical field against women of color, specifically black women, are rampant and sometimes life-threatening for those individuals. These biases are certainly not limited to the medical arena and are rather a function of societal prejudices which maintain racial inequalities within sexual health care.

One clear cut example of this is the way we talk about white female sexuality versus female of colors' sexualities.

According to Sharon Lamb, Tangela Roberts, and Aleksandra Plocha, authors of *Girls of Color, Sexuality, and Sex Education*, while promiscuity in white girls is often excused as a result of trauma and casual sexual activity is viewed as a cry for sexual freedom, sexual activity and expression in black girls is often perceived as an inevitable consequence of "some innate and animalistic oversexualization."[273] Latinas are often characterized in a similar racialized rhetoric of hyper-sexualization which paints them as, "hot-blooded, passionate, teasing, and flirtatious."[274]

As a result, the research and education on the sexual development of girls of color is almost entirely centered around fear-based and risk-based messages, like pregnancy, STIs, and abuse, positioning girls of color as "oversexed and in danger."[275]

For black girls in particular, the overwhelming stance of risk-based sexual development literature and the central focus of sexual education signals to them that being black in America means they are constantly going to be viewed as a problem.[276] White guilt and justification for the horrific abuse and rape of black slaves roots itself in these damaging myths of black promiscuity and high pain tolerances, allowing them to persist.[277]

These stereotypes further diminish the already belittled space female sexuality and sexual health takes up in our society. When girls of color are routinely taught they are

---

273 Sharon Lamb, Tangela Roberts, and Aleksandra Plocha, *Girls of Color, Sexuality, and Sex Education* (New York: Palgrave Macmillan, 2016), 4.

274 Jorge A. Jimenez and José M. Abreu, "Race and sex effects on attitudinal perceptions of acquaintance rape," *Journal of Counseling Psychology* 50, no. 2 (2003), quoted in Sharon Lamb, Tangela Roberts, and Aleksandra Plocha, *Girls of Color, Sexuality, and Sex Education* (New York: Palgrave Macmillan, 2016), 6.

275 Lamb et al., *Girls of Color*, 3.

276 Lamb et al., *Girls of Color*, 3; Melissa V. Harris-Perry, *Sister Citizen: Shame, Stereotypes, and Black Women in America* (New Haven: Yale University Press, 2011), 170.

277 Lamb et al., *Girls of Color*, 3; Linda Villarosa, "Myths about physical racial differences were used to justify slavery — and are still believed by doctors today," *The New York Times Magazine*, August 14, 2019.

more sexually precocious, more likely to get pregnant, and just more innately problematic than white girls, their sexual autonomy and ability to view their sexuality in a healthy, positive light is severely hindered.

Additionally, Lamb et al. notes girls of color who identify as queer, bi, or lesbian are "doubly marked by sexuality" and "defined by her sexual practice" more so than heterosexual girls of color.[278]

This is due to the added layer of sexualization the LGBTQ+ community faces. The sexual objectification of women suffused within our cultural landscape particularly codifies queer women and their sexuality as instruments to further excite and entertain straight men.

Popular tropes in the cultural portrayal of lesbians pandering to the "male gaze" consistently conform to the idea a woman's sexuality exists for men to appropriate and dominate.[279]

> The "male gaze," a term coined by film critic Laura Mulvey, is the act of presenting women from a masculine, heterosexual perspective representing women as sexual objects for the pleasure of the male viewer.[280]

For instance, depictions of lesbian relationships synonymous with "girl-on-girl" pornography satisfy the targeted

---

278 Lamb et al., Girls of Color, 2.
279 Julie Scanlon and Ruth Lewis, "Whose Sexuality Is It Anyway? Women's Experiences of Viewing Lesbians on Screen," Feminist Media Studies 17, no. 6 (2017): 1005, 1007.
280 Dictionary.com, s.v. "male gaze," accessed September 9, 2020; Eva-Maria Jacobsson, A Female Gaze? (Stockholm, Sweden: KTH Royal Institute of Technology, 1999), 7, accessed September 9, 2020.

heterosexual male audience's fantasy of "watching two women make love" (enjoyed by 82.1 percent of men and ranked number six of fifty-five fantasies).[281] Mainstream media packaging over-sexualized and objectifying portrayals of queer women for mass consumption undermines female sexuality outside of heteronormative standards and cements those messages into the cultural understanding of the LGBTQ+ community.

Internalized heteronormative ideals then translate into sexual orientation bias in the medical field. According to a 2015 study based on data from the Sexually Implicit Assessment Test (IAT), heterosexual health care providers implicitly favored heterosexual patients over gay and lesbian patients, and another IAT study found 38 percent of lesbian and gay people favored heterosexual people.[282]

Implicit biases can negatively impact patient-provider relations, especially if the provider plays into damaging stereotypes about the LGBTQ+ community, further internalizing those negative messages and diminishing trust in the provider.

---

281 Christian C. Joyal, Amelie Cossette, and Vanessa LaPierre, "What is an unusual sexual fantasy?" *Journal of Sexual Medicine* 12 (2015): 334, 335, quoted in Julie Scanlon and Ruth Lewis, "Whose Sexuality Is It Anyway? Women's Experiences of Viewing Lesbians on Screen," *Feminist Media Studies* 17, no. 6 (2017): 1008.

282 Michal J. McDowell and Iman K. Berrahou, *Learning to Address Implicit Bias Towards LGBTQ Patients:Case Scenarios* (Boston, MA: National LGBT Health Education Center, 2018), 1. Accessed April 26, 2020; Janice A. Sabin, Rachel G. Riskind, and Brian A. Nosek, "Health Care Providers' Implicit and Explicit Attitudes Toward Lesbian Women and Gay Men," *American Journal of Public Health* 105, no. 9 (September 2015): 1831; John T. Jost, Mahzarin R. Banaji and Brian A. Nosek, "A Decade of System Justification Theory: Accumulated Evidence of Conscious and Unconscious Bolstering of the Status Quo," *Political Psychology* 25, no. 6 (December 2004): 899.

Meg-John (MJ) Barker, an author and former psychotherapist specializing in sex, gender, and relationships, argues these implicit biases can be even worse for bisexual individuals because sexuality is often viewed as binary: you're either straight or gay.

"So, anyone who doesn't fit in to just straight or gay is seen as more suspicious," MJ argues, "and there's this idea bisexuality is just a phase, or bisexual people are a bit dangerous and threatening, and bi people often have to come out repeatedly, because people will assume they're gay or straight depending on their partner. So, there's this extra layer of the everyday challenge of having to constantly make yourself visible. And to be constantly dismissed and questioned, and to receive skepticism from others about your identity, really takes a toll on mental health."

Consequently, bisexual individuals have even greater mental health issues than lesbians or gay men, with only 5 percent of bi youth in a recent Human Rights Campaign survey reporting being "very happy." Additionally, the survey found only 44 percent of bi youth had an adult they could turn to, compared to 54 percent for lesbian and gay youth, and 79 percent of non-LGBT respondents.[283]

Bisexual people are also at a high risk of domestic violence due to their sexual orientation. MJ says people's bisexuality can be used against them in relationships because they are viewed as more suspicious and threatening, and therefore need to be reined in.

---

283 "Bisexual Health Awareness Month: Mental Health in the Bisexual Community," Human Rights Campaign, March 24, 2017.

The stigmas surrounding the bi community bleed into the medical field and disrupt practitioners' perceptions about their patients.

"Bi people are more likely to be labeled with borderline personality disorder," MJ notes, "because if you look at the categories of that disorder, they fit quite a lot of stereotypes of bisexuality. So, bisexual people are more likely to be pathologized by health care professionals."

If we put that in the context of female sexual health issues, like PMDD or vulvar pain, which are so often mischaracterized as mental health conditions or as psychosomatic, it becomes evidently clear bisexual individuals may face additional scrutiny and skepticism from medical providers.

Individuals who don't identify along a sexuality binary, as well as a gender binary, are even further misunderstood by the medical community.

***

Meg-John identifies sexually as bisexual, and gender-wise as non-binary.

> Non-binary and genderqueer (NBGQ) is a general term to describe someone who, "may experience a gender identity that is neither exclusively male or female or is in between or beyond both genders."[284]

---

284 Mairéad Losty and John O'Connor, "Falling outside of the 'nice little binary box': a psychoanalytic exploration of the non-binary gender identity," *Psychoanalytic Psychotherapy* 32, no. 1 (October 2017): 40.

Non-binary is often used as a catch-all term for individuals who identify outside of the strictly binary genders—male and female—and may include those who identify as:

- agender
- bigender
- gender fluid
- genderqueer
- third gender
- or another gender entirely.[285]

When MJ came out as non-binary, they thought it would be similar to when they came out as bisexual years before. But while sexuality isn't something you constantly have to talk about or be reminded of, gender identity is something more immediately flagged in general, everyday interactions.

"You can't get through the day without having to choose which public toilet to go in, or having somebody calling you sir or madam," MJ explains, "so, it's just that much more in your face. People have described it a bit like getting one hundred paper cuts every day because of that sense of constantly being misgendered or having to face that decision of, 'Do you tell people that you're non-binary?' But then they might discriminate against you or be violent toward you. Or, do you let it slide, but then you're invisible, and you're kind of being inauthentic."

Although non-binary and trans individuals both fall outside of the gender binary norm, NBGQ individuals experience

---

285 Elizabeth Boskey, "What Does It Mean to Be Non-Binary or Have Non-Binary Gender?" Very Well Mind, September 28, 2019.

specific health care needs and disparities compared to binary transgender (BT) people (trans women and trans men).[286]

Several studies indicate in the US and UK, NBGQ individuals reported lower qualities of life and higher levels of serious psychological distress than BT and cisgender people.[287] Additionally, although 70 percent of NBGQ individuals indicated a need for gender-related counseling, only 31 percent had access to psychological clinical services, compared to 73 percent of BT individuals.[288] This disparity could stem from concerns that mental and medical health providers are unfamiliar with NBGQ health needs and identity, as they are often misgendered or addressed from a binary concept of trans identity.[289]

When MJ goes to the doctor, there is never a box or a space for their gender identity, and their gender has been consistently misread and misunderstood by practitioners. Yet, despite these obstacles, MJ's path of recognizing their gender and

---

286 Cristiano Scandurra et al., "Health of Non-binary and Genderqueer People: A Systematic Review," *Frontiers in Psychology* 10, no. 1453 (June 2019): 1.

287 Scandurra et al., "Health of Non-binary," 2; Sandy E. James et al., *The Report of the 2015 U.S. Transgender Survey.* (Washington, DC: National Center for Transgender Equality, 2016), 105. Accessed June 8, 2020.

288 Scandurra et al., "Health of Non-binary," 2; Sandy E. James et al., *The Report of the 2015*, 99.

289 Scandurra et al., "Health of Non-binary," 2; James E. Lykens, Allen J. LeBlanc, and Walter O. Bockting, "Healthcare Experiences Among Young Adults Who Identify as Genderqueer or Nonbinary," *LGBT Health* 5, no. 3 (April 2018): 191; Aleta Baldwin et al., "Transgender and Genderqueer Individuals› Experiences with Health Care Providers: What›s Working, What›s Not, and Where Do We Go from Here?" *Journal of Health Care for the Poor and Underserved* 29, no. 4 (November 2018): 1300.

sexual identity helped to free themselves of other burdens negatively impacting their sexual health.

"I definitely always had this sense of being attracted to more than one gender, and that my gender didn't fit neatly into the boxes of male or female," MJ says. Growing up as a socialized female, and especially working as a sex therapist with women clients, MJ was all too familiar with the negative aspects of female socialization and stereotypes.

"I saw so many of [my clients] were having so much unwanted sex," MJ says, "because they felt like they had to have sex in order to please a partner, be more desirable, or keep a partner, which is still such a strong message women get: you have to have sex in order to remain in the relationship, and your main job in life is to have a relationship, so you better keep doing it, you know? Certainly, once you've got kids, as well. That's your job—to keep the family together."

MJ felt they were being squished into these restrictive gender binary rules as a socialized female and realized they were having unwanted sex and prioritizing the pleasure of *other* people and being desirable for *other* people, more so than doing what was best for themselves.

MJ's journey toward identifying as non-binary was strongly influenced by the negative impact gendered rules were having on their relationships and their sense of sexuality and self.

This mentality feeds into MJ's work and theory on relationships today and dismantling sexuality norms that present

Western understandings of white, cisgendered, heterosexual relationships and sex as the ideal. MJ argues:

"We're coming from this incorrect starting point, which is to start with the norm, and then try and get people to fit that law, or maybe expand out of that norm slightly. It's almost like we need to start from a completely different place, which is to question all of the cultural messages people receive about sex, to help them really tune into themselves and communicate with others and to make consent. And consent is just so much more than somebody getting a 'yes' or 'no' to a particular sex act. We have to be mindful of power, we have to be mindful of the cultural scripts people feel they have to follow. We have to be mindful that a lot of people are conditioned into being enthusiastic toward things they're not really enthusiastic toward, like women's socialization, which mainly puts them in a place where they're expected to be enthusiastic about things they really don't want to do."

Deconstructing gender norms is a crucial step in the right direction. We have to reexamine the conversation as it relates to female pain and consent. We have to look at all of the restrictive social rules disempowering women and AFAB individuals when it comes to embracing sexuality or seeking sexual health care.

Expanding beyond these concerns, we also have to understand all of the other inhibiting factors—homophobia, racism, ableism, etc.—which can not only physically prevent someone from obtaining sexual health care, but also devalue the importance of their sexuality and right to sexual freedoms.

CHAPTER 13

But, Have You Tried Lube?

"If I were a patient with no knowledge, I would find it extremely overwhelming." This is a quote from Dr. Jen Chu, a women's health specialist and physical therapist who has made it her life's mission to ensure her patients never feel this way at her practice.

Tinkling bells greet visitors as they enter the Individualized Therapeutic Rehabilitation (ITR) Physical Therapy office. The space is small, with two private rooms in the back for sessions and a waiting area supplied with water and health magazines for patients. It is a quiet space filled with the sound of waves crashing from a small white noise machine. The space, intentionally or not, speaks to the environment Jen envisioned for her practice when she founded ITR back in 2001: quality, specialized, and supportive one-on-one care for every patient.

When she first started out as a physical therapist in the late 90s, a recent college graduate eager to employ her hard-earned skills, Jen found herself struggling to embrace the workplace culture. Unfortunately, it was a time when larger hospital systems were supplanting mom-and-pop shops, insurance companies were cracking down on reimbursement claims, and physical therapy jobs were in short supply.

Jen's days were filled with more patients than she could handle, often requiring her to treat five or six orthopedic patients at a time to make up for the hour-long time slots she had to block off for women's-health-based patients. Rushing around treating as many patients as possible to meet her clinic's billing demands with little emphasis placed on the quality or thoughtfulness of the care did not sit well for Jen.

"After almost five years, I felt burnt out and I didn't like what I was doing. I didn't," she says. "It just didn't feel right. I just felt like patients deserved one-on-one quality care."

Nearly twenty years later, Jen has succeeded in making this simple mission come true, and ITR has grown to include five other PTs, joining the ranks of a myriad of other PT offices in the greater DC area. But to get to where she is today required heaps of effort and dedication just to convince physicians she can offer beneficial adjunct services to their patients suffering from chronic pain.

Using manual therapy to treat chronic pain is still a relatively new technique which is not yet mainstream, especially when it comes to treating sexual dysfunction in women.

> *Sexual dysfunction comprises persistent, recurrent problems with sexual response, desire, orgasm, or pain that distresses you or strains your relationship with your partner.*[290]

---

290 "Female Sexual Dysfunction," Mayo Clinic, Accessed September 12, 2020.

Disruption of any component involved in sexual response (physiology, emotions, experiences, beliefs, lifestyle and relationships) can impact sexual desire and lead to symptoms of sexual dysfunction, including:

- low sexual desire
- sexual arousal disorder
- orgasmic disorder
- and sexual pain disorder.[291]

Despite the fact female sexual dysfunction (FSD) afflicts approximately 40 percent of women, including it as a part of women's overall sexual health in the medical sphere is still a wildly new concept.[292]

The women's sexual health movement really only came into force during the 1960s, gaining momentum during the 70s before hitting several roadblocks when Reagan sailed into office in 1981.[293]

In the beginning, women fought to gain control over their basic reproductive rights:

- the right to safe and legal abortions
- access to birth control

---

291 Ibid.

292 Kyan J. Allahdadi, Rita C.A. Tostes, and R. Clinton Webb, "Female Sexual Dysfunction: Therapeutic Options and Experimental Challenges," *Cardiovasc Hematol Agents Med Chem* 7, no. 4 (October 2009): 260.

293 Francine H. Nichols, "History of the Women's Health Movement in the 20th Century," *Journal of Obstetric, Gynecologic, & Neonatal Nursing* 29, no. 1 (June 1999): 56-57.

- authority over their body during childbirth
- and access to accurate information and medical care.[294]

Nearly sixty years later, though we've made progress on many of these issues, we are still fighting some of the same battles for the same basic rights women were fighting for (and won in some cases!) back in the 60s. So, it's not hard to imagine addressing women's sexual health needs outside of sexually transmitted diseases (STDs), contraceptives, and pregnancy is not common practice.

Consequently, we're left with a women's health care scene equivalent to a "patchwork quilt with gaps" well into the twenty-first century, alluding to the separation between specialties, oftentimes functioning in isolation.[295] Specialists like Jen are working to bridge the gap to expand beyond the borders of traditional discipline practice.

"I've been in this role for a long time," Jen comments, "so I've seen some really positive changes. But I also believe the ball is just starting to roll downhill. We were for a really long time trying to roll the ball up."

Though we have come a long way, it does feel in many respects like we are still pushing hard to roll that ball up. Part of the issue stems from physicians themselves refusing to believe a

---

294 Nichols, "History of the Women's," 56, 57, 59, 61.
295 Carolyn M. Clancy and Charlea T. Massion, "American Women's Health Care: A Patchwork Quilt With Gaps," *JAMA* 268, no. 14 (1992), quoted in Pamela Karney, "Women's Health: An Evolving Mosaic," *Journal of General Internal Medicine* 15, no. 8 (August 2000): 600.

woman when she says she is in pain, or having complications, or just that something feels off. There is often a tendency for doctors dealing with female sexual health to minimize their concerns and chalk their pain up to "normal womanly processes."

When Jen first opened ITR, she remembers a patient one day expressing concern over incessant pain in her pelvic area. As Jen began her examination, the patient continued, "My doctor says it's all in my head. I don't know, though, it feels like more than that and I wanted to see if you could help."

Jen's eyes flashed at the asinine assumption her patient's pain was simply imagined or intangible and replied empathetically, "Of course it's not only in your head! There are physical things going on with your body. I'll show you."

Resuming the examination, Jen gently palpated trigger points in the patient's external pelvic floor muscles to check for areas of pain. Discovering a spot of concern, she asked, "Feel that? That's tight muscle, that's a physical trigger point right there."

She desperately wanted to validate her patient, to show them there were physical expressions of their pain rooted in their body. Over the years she encountered countless other patients who had been holding onto pain for decades and had been to doctor after doctor after doctor who told them to take Advil or drink a glass of wine or use more lubricant.

"I mean, most of my patients could swim in a tub of lubricant and it's just not—it's not the problem."

On the contrary, throughout her work in physical therapy and as a mind and body coach, Jen has come to understand our bodies hold negative energy and trauma and those emotions not only present as depression and anxiety, but also manifest physically as pain. So, trauma, which can come from abuse or assault can also come from any suppressed negative emotion, sends messages to our bodies.

Those messages will build and build and build, Jen explains, "and will begin to scream until they are heard. Until we have no choice but to listen as our bodies begin to break down."

Jen likes to say there's a reason we have the saying, "Listen to your gut." She argues our bodies are immensely intelligent and if we were taught to listen to what they are telling us rather than ignore or quash those signs, we could change the face of how we treat chronic pain.

Imagine living with chronic pain for years, feeling hopeless after every doctor you visit can't help you with your invisible affliction, and finally arriving at a specialized physical therapy clinic. When you show up for your appointment, instead of lying down on the table and saying for the thousandth time, "I have pain. Fix me," your therapist tells you that you have the power, with their guidance and expertise, to treat your pain by listening to your own innate intelligence to identify how your mental innerworkings may be triggering physical responses.

Suddenly, the patient becomes empowered to take their healing journey into their own hands; their pain is not only validated, it is understood.

But listening to your gut is often much more difficult when the subject is sexual pain and dysfunction. As young children, we tend to receive messages it is objectionable to express unpleasant emotions, particularly with anything surrounding sexuality or puberty or our bodies.

Jen herself received these messages growing up in a Catholic family. While she was never taught sexuality was wrong, her family generally avoided the subject. But even merely ignoring the topic can push ideas of shame and secrecy regarding sexual health on a child, causing them to lock those feelings deep down with no healthy way out.

Moreover, when we as women are instructed to act lady-like, to be polite, to avoid being "too emotional," we are more likely to disregard the more uncomfortable topic of our sexual health. In doing so, we fail to honor an integral part of who we are, harboring instead destructive feelings of shame and self-loathing, especially when we face complications.

We live our lives feeling incomplete, broken, and not wholly healthy. Also, we perpetuate this culture which allows unmistakable pain to go unnoticed and model it for the next generation.

"So all that's going to happen," Jen argues, "is they're going to grow up the same way, having very similar feelings—being embarrassed about their own bodies, being embarrassed to touch themselves, being embarrassed to tap into what they feel and when that happens, it's going to come out sideways."

So, yes, it's uncomfortable; luckily, we have people like Jen who are working hard every day to use their expertise to provide an invaluable resource to people who are tired of allowing their pain to rule their lives. She, and other specialists like her, are often literal saviors to women who have never before heard their concerns legitimized, much less fully supported.

The hope is these women can then become their own advocates, reassuring themselves they are not their pain and they have every right to seek medical and emotional help. Receiving professional services which yield tangible, life-changing results is so empowering it could prove positive for wider advocacy movements that help reach those who have yet to seek these resources.

CHAPTER 14

Shameless

Dr. Jennifer Lincoln, an opinionated, take-no-bullshit kind of person and doctor, is everything that's right when it comes to the field of female sexual health. Trained in a progressive program at the Oregon Health and Science University in Portland, Oregon, Dr. Jennifer had exposure to a full spectrum of women's health care.

She had experts in vulvar issues like lichen sclerosus, vestibulitis, vulvodynia, and other chronic issues in her residency program.

She had some of the best pelvic floor therapists at her disposal to treat conditions such as vaginismus or pelvic sexual health disorders during her training.

She developed her medical skills and knowledge in an environment which exuded respect for the women they were treating and stressed the importance of removing all shame from the patient-doctor equation.

Dr. Jennifer is now a practicing OB Hospitalist in Portland, Oregon who strives to bring her patients the best care possible. She is a testament to what comprehensive sexual health education can promote in her field. As a woman, she is of course privy to the backward, hypocritical, and often demoralizing expectations and constraints our society places on females. As a medical provider, she sees how these standards can play out to the detriment of a woman's health and well-being.

"I think being in this field, and seeing what we see every day— hearing women's stories about how they had been abused or how they had been raped or how they had been treated a certain way because their doctor didn't believe in birth control or abortion, or how they have been blown off by people because they're a woman and they just were told to deal with their heavy periods—it really opened my eyes to how much politics and stereotypes go into putting up barriers in the office, and even before the woman gets to the office," Jennifer says.

One such barrier so often presenting itself in the office is doctors shaming women for anything from their shaving habits to their sexual preferences.

Jennifer has had women come to her whose previous doctors have made fun of them, made them feel stupid, disrespected their wishes, invalidated their concerns, and more. She argues any type of shaming is completely counterproductive and offensive because "once we put our judgment in there, women are not going to be honest with us. And the second you begin to judge you're telling a woman she can't tell you anything because you've already decided what kind of person she is."

That kind of negative scrutiny can be incredibly damaging to a person's self-image, not to mention threatening to her overall health.

"It's a form of abuse," Jennifer says, as shaming violates the patient-doctor trust needed for patients to feel comfortable and doctors to do their job correctly. Arguably, if an OB/GYN or other medical professionals cannot provide unbiased information and an unconditionally supportive environment for their patients, then they need to decide if what they're doing is really what is best for their patients.

"We cannot be setting up roadblocks based on our personal judgments," stresses Jennifer.

Doctors have a responsibility to be as open, understanding, and knowledgeable as possible to help break down any barriers and provide their patients with the care they need. Jennifer also underscores the importance of educating our doctors because if they don't know an issue or condition exists, how are they going to accurately diagnose and treat their patient? This is a large reason why so many chronic vaginal issues, especially "invisible" conditions, go undiagnosed and untreated for years.

In Jennifer's case, she was fortunate to have such an all-encompassing education and residency track. She is fortunate now to work in an area home to some amazing women's health specialists to whom she can refer her patients because there are so many women in the US who are missed or dismissed by our medical system.

"I think about the average woman in rural America who has to travel twenty or thirty miles to even get to a gynecologist," Jen points out, "and then if that woman needs specialist care, her gynecologist might not even know where to find that or how to send her to that."

For doctors without the scope of Jennifer's training, it becomes easier to dredge up some internalized messages about women's sexual health and sexuality, because these practitioners don't know where to look for further information or don't know where to refer patients.

"When it comes to women's sexual health issues, we are notorious for telling women, 'Oh well you know, that's just how women are, and men are the ones who want to have sex. You have vaginal dryness? You just have to deal with it. Sex should hurt—you just have to relax, maybe try having a glass of wine.' We just push so many things under the rug and then women internalize that, and they think it's just them."

Beyond inadequate training on women's health issues, doctor's may further fail their patients if they do not ask the right kind of questions during an appointment, consultation, or exam. Oftentimes, discovering underlying issues which do fall under the umbrella of "normal womanly processes" still requires physicians to dig deeper than the surface-level questions of, "Are you currently sexually active with men, women, or both?"

Women are constantly taught to just smile and pretend everything's fine, to not make a big deal out of nothing, to avoid dramatics. These issues can feel embarrassing and shameful, especially in the context of a society which does not allow women to comfortably or openly discuss anything related to their sexual health.

So, even if it seems or looks as though nothing is amiss, it's important for medical professionals to stop and ask their patients probing questions:

- Are you experiencing any pain?
- Are you having particularly difficult periods?
- Are you experiencing any symptoms which could be warning signs for a bigger issue?

Without guiding questions, many women will not bring those problems up on their own.

Jennifer has had many experiences with women coming to her with issues they knew they had but couldn't find anyone else to help or believe them, or who didn't even know their condition had a name.

A patient came to her once complaining of pain in their vagina. After questioning them further, Jennifer found the patient couldn't have sex without excruciating pain and couldn't have a Pap smear done because the speculum was too painful.

The patient was told by previous physicians they just needed to relax and pain during sex was normal for women.

Even before performing a quick physical examination of the patient, Jennifer had an idea she was dealing with levator myalgia or pelvic floor dysfunction. At this point, Jennifer was a little aghast because it is the "most basic of exams to be able to assess a woman's pelvic floor muscles and feel they are tight as rubber bands and know their pelvic floor is obviously in a state of complete contraction and dysfunction."

It was disconcerting for her to realize other OB/GYNs would not recognize this very palpable condition which is easily treatable with the appropriate therapy.

For Jennifer, it was no issue. She quickly diagnosed the patient and without hesitation gave them concrete next steps:

"I've got this pelvic floor physical therapist who works two floors down and I want you to go work with her and we're going to do some dilator work and we're going to prescribe you some topical lidocaine so you can even deal with the touch, since you've got some vulva issues as well."

Jennifer says afterwards her patient just broke down crying, partly from relief because they hadn't realized there was a fix for their issues, and partly from anger because it took so long for them to get any answer at all. Once they found a doctor who actually listened and who was properly educated, the solution—overlooked by every other doctor—was easy and straightforward.

"If you don't know it exists, you're not going to look for it. You're just going to tell a woman, 'Oh just deal with it.' It's been very satisfying to feel like you're connecting the dots and helping these people. But at the same time," Jennifer huffs, "like, why is this not part of common doctor knowledge?"

In an effort to close this gap in education, Jennifer has taken to social media to post informative bits of advice or to dispel common myths about female sexual health. She posts regularly for her more than sixty thousand followers on Instagram and more than one million followers on TikTok in an effort to make this information more accessible to as many people as possible. She hopes by publicly sharing this information herself as a credible source, women will realize it's not just in their head, they shouldn't have to put up with someone telling them to just deal with it, and hopefully will feel empowered to speak up to their doctors about their issues.

Jennifer is intent on giving women their power back, power which has been stripped away from them, in any way possible. She feels like part of her job is "calling out the bullshit of women's health in America," a sentiment reiterated by many other OB/GYNs she knows. She is here to do more than prescribe birth control or deliver a baby; she is here to treat the whole woman, including the societal issues inherent in the environment within which women exist.

Jennifer loves what she does, and she appreciates the unique intimacy that comes with her job, and the additional responsibility to do her job well. She can only hope others in her field will progress toward a more informed, understanding, and supportive approach to female sexual health.

Conclusion

My hope is this book will both lend itself to disrupting the current thought process when it comes to sex and female bodies and provide some insight into *why* we need to stop conflating female sexual/reproductive systems and pain. At the end of the day, the core idea with which we all have to reconcile is women and AFAB people deserve sexual autonomy. It seems simple to say, but our country and our society remains so far removed from realizing this.

Achieving true sexual liberation for everyone regardless of sex, gender, race, ability, etc., requires individuals to unpack personal implicit biases. This feeds into a slew of issues: educators teaching comprehensive sex education, doctors validating every patient's concerns, researchers putting more resources into understudied health care issues and intersections, authors and artists and tv producers creating content which more widely represents sexual experiences, and governments passing laws and implementing policies protecting and aiding vulnerable populations in the sexual health and sexuality sphere.

These are the shifts in culture and advances in society any progressive movement or ideology wants to see, but as we all know, they don't happen overnight.

This book is not meant to be an exhaustive examination of all the overlooked sexual health and sexuality issues women and AFAB individuals face. It is merely a continuation of conversations surrounding sex positivity and healthy sex behaviors so maybe the people dealing with these issues feel a little less alone. Maybe it will introduce someone else to a new concept or idea they had never before considered. Maybe it will help all of us become a little less uncomfortable saying the words "sex" and "vagina" and "period."

We often use this allegory or phrase of "get the ball rolling" in reference to starting something. But we tend to think the hardest part is the initial push of the ball, and afterward inertia or gravity takes over. With any social movement, though, that ball is not rolling without the force of friction slowing it down, and it's not rolling down a steep, clear hill. It's constantly getting hung up on roots and boulders and plateaus. If we really want to see change, we have to take it one step at a time. A nudge here, a shove there to help the ball, and this movement, continue its journey.

This requires each and every one of us to ask ourselves, and others, questions which open up new avenues of thought and uncover the preconceived notions hindering change.

Why do we think ignoring things that make us uncomfortable, skirting around the messy bits and sloppily fumbling for the right words, benefits anyone?

Why is it there are certain parts of our bodies we feel we can't talk to our doctors about?

Why is it there are certain parts of our bodies our doctors give less attention to?

How is it everyone is talking about sex all the time without actually ever talking about it?

If we continue to treat sex as this big scary thing, confusing it with sin or drenching it in a discourse of shame, young people are going to continue to grow up thinking sex is something they shouldn't talk about openly and honestly. When we talk about sex as shameful or dirty, or chiefly focus on its negative aspects, we teach people it's ok to shame others about sex. When we teach some groups of people sexual activity is a form of natural sexual liberation and tell others it's wanton, we create a predatory environment. Adolescents well into adulthood internalize those messages and cope by making jokes or engaging in risky sexual behavior in rebellion, or in the name of "sexual liberation."

Because their sexual health has never actually been a priority—they're just following the norms for what society *thinks* is best for their sexual health.

And when those messages are, "female sexual health is not a priority" and "female sexual expression is immoral," we end up with a gap in research on female sexual health issues, doctors who cannot or will not believe, protect, and treat their patients, and women and AFAB individuals who don't know how to talk about their bodies, can't find answers, and feel broken.

We cannot continue promoting the limited view we currently hold of sexual development, sexual health, sex, and sexuality.

Not only does this perpetuate many common female sexual health issues, in some cases, it can be the very cause of their existence. Understanding these issues, stigmas, and systemic barriers will improve the physical and emotional health of millions of women and AFAB individuals in the US, and millions more in generations to come.

Acknowledgments

Along this book-writing journey, I have had the opportunity to talk to, reconnect with, and learn from so many different people. Writing and publishing a book is not a one-woman job, and I am so grateful for all the time, support, and commitment my contributors have shown me along the way. Fulfilling this goal would not have been possible without you.

Thank you first and foremost to my family and friends for supporting me through every step of this process. Thank you to my mom and dad for immediately jumping on board when I said I wanted to write a book and for your constant encouragement. Thank you to all my friends for listening to me talk about the ups and downs of this long journey and for sharing in this experience with me.

Thank you to my editors Jordan Waterwash, Jen Wichman, and Kendra Kadam, as well as Eric Koester, Brian Bies, and New Degree Press, for making this book a reality.

Thank you to all my interviewees for taking time out of your busy schedules to talk with me and share your stories. You helped bring life, intimacy, and vulnerability to this book. Thank you to the following individuals, and to those who have chosen to remain anonymous, for your bravery in speaking out about these issues:

Elizabeth Wright
Caroline Miani
Trista Marie McGovern
Morgan Givens
Laura Kiesel
Meg-John Barker
Jennifer Chu
Jennifer Lincoln
Les Henderson
Tangela Roberts
Sigmund Hough
Zoë Peterson
Mira Scarnecchia
Naomi Jackson
Annet Dragavon
Morgan Sheets
Sarah Soliman
Brandy Plott
Cheryl Morris
Allison Landry

Also, thank you to everyone who pre-ordered the eBook, paperback, and multiple copies to make publishing possible, and who helped spread the word about *My Venus Flytrap Won't Open* to gather amazing momentum and help me publish a book I am proud of. I am sincerely grateful for all of your help:

Peter Dore
Kathryn Morgan

Hannah Hembree
Mara McDonough
Samantha Miller
Dory Freeman
Morgan McKeown
Sarah Johnson
Laura Hamilton
Angie Dierks
Maia Anderson
Lexie Jamieson
Daniel Herschlag
Elizabeth McKendry
Tyler Sanders
Zainab Mirza
Judy Harrison*
Dan Harrison*
Marieme Ba
Kylie Greenleaf
Lucy LaCasse*
Jennifer McKendry
Emma Hartl
Daniel Acosta Rivas
Abigail Cassada
Taylor Marinko
Alice Turner
Trudy Harrison
Jessica Foster
Casey Bitner
Paul Wapner
Charlotte Turner
Brandan Persaud*
Faith Lewis

Julie Harrison*
Mira Scarnecchia
Julie Dumais
Michaela Rutschow
K. Gulrich
Kimberly Walsh
Jenna Block
Donna Cassada
Monica Gunkle*
Karen Friedman
Emily Lytle
Elizabeth Wright
Bert Follansbee
Debra McDonough
Kay Whitmore
Katy Jutras
J. L. Caven
Carly Milkowski
Julia Steinbach
Linda Labbe
Laurie Palow
David Qui*
Erin MacDonald
Julia Lazarek
Donna Snyder*
Lisa Bridgham
Jake Swanson
Samantha Haquia
Eliza Palow
Allison Johntry
Ian Engelman
Gwyneth Barry

Jessie Mehrhoff
Brian Dumais*
Constance Ortolani
Jillian McCarthy
Jacquie Dore*
Emma Koukos
Dana Ricker
Zachary Samalonis
Luke Barcy
Donald Watson*
Kimberly Cassada
Kristy Peng
Morgan Maddock
Sarah Lyon
Dennis Manzer
Lillian Menkens-Weiler
Emily Michels
Judy Burakowski*
Susie Gravel
Jim Vogel*
Maggie D'Andrea
Terese King*
Jill Clancy
Emma Freeman
Larry Dore
Tessa Wright
Tracey Dubois
Kathy Neddeau*
Denise Couture
Katie Barker
Elliot Dumais
Susan Haversat

Madeleine Dumais
Katherine Ruff
Anne Ball
Jane Palmer
Jon York
Jeff Dumais
Lincoln MacIsaac
Christopher Niebuhr
Tina Veilleux
Kimberly Bridgham*

APPENDIX

Introduction

- Brown, Theodore, and Elizabeth Fee. "Alfred C. Kinsey: A Pioneer Of Sex Research." *American journal of public health* 93, no. 6 (June 2003): 896-897. https://doi.org/10.2105/ajph.93.6.896.

- Geary, M.S. "An analysis of the women's health movement and its impact on the delivery of health care within the United States." *Nurse Practitioner* 20, no. 11 PT 1 (1995): 24-27. https://pubmed.ncbi.nlm.nih.gov/8587743/.

- Nichols, Francine. "History of the Women's Health Movement in the 20ᵗʰ Century." *Journal of Obstetric, Gynecologic & Neonatal Nursing* 29, no. 1 (June 1999): 56-64. https://doi.org/10.1111/j.1552-6909.2000.tb02756.x *Science and Its Times: Understanding the Social Significance of Scientific Discovery,* s.v. "The Study of Human Sexuality." Accessed August 21, 2020, https://www.encyclopedia.com/science/encyclopedias-almanacs-transcripts-and-maps/study-human-sexuality.

- Wardell, D. "Margaret Sanger: birth control's successful revolutionary." *American journal of public health* 70, no. 7 (July 1980): 736-742. https://doi.org/10.2105/AJPH.70.7.736.

Chapter 1

- American Social Hygiene Association. *The Case Against the Red Light.* New York: United States Public Health Service, 1920. Box 54, Folder "Social Hygiene," Adèle Goodman Clark papers 1849-1978, VCU Libraries Gallery. https://gallery.library.vcu.edu/items/show/82552.

- Andrinopoulos, Katherine, Deanna Kerrigan, and Jonathan M. Ellen. "Understanding Sex Partner Selection From the Perspective of Inner-City Black Adolescents." *Perspectives on Sexual and Reproductive Health* 38, no. 3 (September 2006): 132-138. https://doi.org/10.1363/3813206.

- Blakemore, Erin. "The Scandalous Sex Parties That Made Americans Hate Flappers." History. Last modified July 21, 2019. https://www.history.com/news/the-scandalous-sex-parties-that-made-americans-hate-flappers.

- Boonstra, Heather D. "Advocates Call for a New Approach After the Era of 'Abstinence-Only' Sex Education." *Guttmacher Policy Review* 12, no. 1 (March 2009): 6-11. https://www.guttmacher.org/gpr/2009/03/advocates-call-new-approach-after-era-abstinence-only-sex-education.

- Brown, Theodore M., and Elizabeth Fee. "Alfred C. Kinsey: A Pioneer Of Sex Research." *American Journal of Public Health* 93, no. 6 (June 2003): 896-897. https://doi.org/10.2105/AJPH.93.6.896.

- Bullock, Darryl W. "Pansy Craze: the wild 1930s drag parties that kickstarted gay nightlife." *The Guardian*, September 14, 2017. https://www.theguardian.com/music/2017/sep/14/pansy-craze-the-wild-1930s-drag-parties-that-kickstarted-gay-nightlife.

- Chen, Emma. "Black Face, Queer Space: The Influence of Black Lesbian & Transgender Blues Women of the Harlem Renaissance on Emerging Queer Communities." *Historical Perspectives: Santa Clara University Undergraduate Journal of History, Series II* 21, no. 8 (2016): 19-29. https://scholarcommons. scu.edu/historical-perspectives/vol21/iss1/8.

- Cohen, Nancy L. *Delirium: The Politics of Sex in America.* Berkley, CA: Counterpoint, 2012.

- Cornblatt, Johannah. "A Brief History of Sex Ed in America." *Newsweek*, October 27, 2009. https://www.newsweek.com/ brief-history-sex-ed-america-81001.

- Davies, Susan L., Ralph J. DiClemente, Gina M. Wingood, Kathy Harrington, Richard A. Crosby, and Kim Oh. "Predictors of Inconsistent Contraceptive Use among Adolescent Girls: Findings from a Prospective Study." *Journal of Adolescent Health* 39, no. 1 (July 2006): 43-49. https://doi.org/10.1016/j. jadohealth.2005.10.011.

- Davis, Angela Y. *Blues Legacies and Black Feminism: Gertrude Ma Rainey, Bessie Smith, and Billie Holiday.* New York: Vintage Books, 1999.

- Department of Justice Bureau of Justice Statistics. "National Crime Victimization Survey 2010-2016." 2017. Cited in Rape, Abuse & Incest National Network. "The Criminal Justice System: Statistics." Accessed August 31, 2020. https://www.rainn. org/statistics/criminal-justice-system.

- *Dictionary.com.* S.v. "gender binary." Accessed September 7, 2020, https://www.dictionary.com/browse/gender-binary.

- Dzhanova, Yelena. "The battle over abortion rights: Here's what's at stake in 2020." CNBC. Last modified January 6, 2020. https://www.cnbc.com/2020/01/06/the-battle-over-abortion-rights-heres-whats-at-stake-in-2020.html.

- Eagle Forum. "Eagle Forum Brochure." Accessed August 31, 2020. https://eagleforum.org/about/brochure.html.

- Elia, John P. "School-Based Sexuality Education: A Century of Sexual and Social Control." In *Sexuality Education - Past Present and Future,* edited by Elizabeth Schroder and Judy Kuriansky, 33-57. Westport, CT: Praeger, 2009.

- *Encyclopedia Britannica Online.* s.v. "Moral Majority." Accessed August 31, 2020. https://www.britannica.com/biography/Paul-Weyrich.

- Frost, Jennifer J. and Anne K. Driscoll. *Sexual and reproductive health of U.S. Latinas: a literature review.* New York: Guttmacher Institute, 2006. Accessed May 30, 2020. https://www.guttmacher.org/sites/default/files/report_pdf/or19.pdf.

- Fullilove, Mindy Thompson, Robert E. Fullilove, III, Katherine Haynes, and Shirley Gross. "Black Women and AIDS Prevention: A View Toward Understanding the Gender Rules." *The Journal of Sex Research* 27, no. 1 (February 1990): 47-64. https://doi.org/10.1080/00224499009551541.

- Gender Spectrum. "Understanding Gender." Accessed September 7, 2020. https://genderspectrum.org/articles/understanding-gender.

- Guttmacher Institute. "Sex and HIV Education." Last modified September 1, 2020. https://www.guttmacher.org/state-policy/explore/sex-and-hiv-education.

- Hall, Kelli S., Jessica M. Sales, Kelli A. Komro, and John Santelli. "The State of Sex Education in the United States" *Journal of Adolescent Health* 58, no. 6 (June 2016): 595-597. https://doi.org/10.1016/j.jadohealth.2016.03.032.

- Hills, Rachel. "What Every Generation Gets Wrong About Sex." *Time*, December 2, 2014. https://time.com/3611781/sexual-revolution-revisited/.

- History. "The Roaring Twenties History." Last modified August 12, 2020. https://www.history.com/topics/roaring-twenties/roaring-twenties-history.

- HIV.gov. "A Timeline of HIV and AIDS." Accessed September 22, 2020. https://www.hiv.gov/hiv-basics/overview/history/hiv-and-aids-timeline.

- Hix, Lisa. "Singing the Lesbian Blues in 1920s Harlem." Collectors Weekly. July 9, 2013. https://www.collectorsweekly.com/articles/singing-the-lesbian-blues-in-1920s-harlem/.

- Holland, Janet, Caroline Ramazanoglu, Sue Scott, Sue Sharpe, and Rachel Thomson."Sex, gender and power: young women's sexuality in the shadow of AIDS," *Sociology of Health & Illness* 12, no. 3 (September 1990): 336-350. https://doi.org/10.1111/1467-9566.ep11347264.

- Intersex Society of North America. "What is intersex?" Accessed September 7, 2020. https://isna.org/faq/what_is_intersex/.

- Jani, Shruti. "Since It's Rubbished So Much, What Exactly Is Sex-Positive Feminism?" Feminism in India. March 27, 2018. https://feminisminindia.com/2018/03/27/sex-positive-feminism-101/.

- Jones, James H. *Alfred C. Kinsey: A Public/Private Life.* New York: W. W. Norton & Company, 1997. Quoted in Theodore M. Brown and Elizabeth Fee. "Alfred C. Kinsey: A Pioneer Of Sex Research." *American Journal of Public Health* 93, no. 6 (June 2003): 896-897. https://doi.org/10.2105/AJPH.93.6.896.

- Kantor, Leslie M., John S. Santelli, Julien Teitler, and Randall Balmer. "Abstinence-only policies and programs: An overview." *Sexuality Research & Social Policy* 5, no.6 (September 2008): 6-17. https://doi.org/10.1525/srsp.2008.5.3.6.

- Kay, Julie F. and Ashley Jackson. *Sex, Lies & Stereotypes: How Abstinence-Only Programs Harm Women and Girls.* New York: Legal Momentum, 2008. Accessed May 30, 2020. http://hrp.law.harvard.edu/wp-content/uploads/2013/03/sexlies_stereotypes2008.pdf.

- Keeping Fit— An Exhibit for Older Boys and Young Men, 10, 1919-1922. Box 171, Folder 8. American Social Health Association Records, University of Minnesota Libraries, Social Welfare History Archives. http://purl.umn.edu/111816.

- Kirby, Douglas. *Emerging Answers 2007: Research Findings on Programs to Reduce Teen Pregnancy and Sexually Transmitted Diseases.* Washington, DC: National Campaign to Prevent Teen and Unplanned Pregnancy, 2007. Accessed May 30, 2020. https://powertodecide.org/sites/default/files/resources/primary-download/emerging-answers.pdf.

- Lawrence, Jill. "Senate Says Federal AIDS Education Material Can't Promote Homosexuality." AP News. October 14, 1987. https://apnews.com/article/65c596e0514c81b20536d9cb-f33c066f.

- *Merriam-Webster.* S.v. "cisgender." Accessed September 7, 2020. https://www.merriam-webster.com/dictionary/cisgender.

- *Merriam-Webster.* S.v. "transgender." Accessed September 7, 2020. https://www.merriam-webster.com/dictionary/transgender.

- National Center for Transgender Equality. "Understanding Non-Binary People: How to Be Respectful and Supportive." October 5, 2018. https://transequality.org/issues/resources/understanding-non-binary-people-how-to-be-respectful-and-supportive.

- Operation Rescue. "Who We Are." Accessed August 31, 2020. https://www.operationrescue.org/about-us/who-we-are/.

- Our Bodies Our Selves. "A Brief History of Birth Control in the U.S." Last modified July 8, 2020. https://www.ourbodiesourselves.org/book-excerpts/health-article/a-brief-history-of-birth-control/.

- *Oxford Reference.* s.v. "gender essentialism." Accessed June 2, 2020. https://www.oxfordreference.com/view/10.1093/oi/authority.20110803095846595.

- Philipson, Robert, dir. *T'ain't nobody's bizness : queer blues divas of the 1920's.* 2011; San Francisco, CA: Shoga Films. DVD.

- Planned Parenthood. "History of Sex Education in the U.S." November 2016, 1-17. https://www.plannedparenthood.org/uploads/filer_public/da/67/da67fd5d-631d-438a-85e8-a446d90fd1e3/20170209_sexed_d04_1.pdf.

- Rowden, Terry. "Harlem Undercover: Difference and Desire in African American Popular Music, 1920-1940." *English Language Notes* 45, no. 2 (October 2007): 23-31. https://doi.org/10.1215/00138282-45.2.23.

- Russell, Stephen T. and Faye C. H. Lee, "Practitioners' Perspectives on Effective Practices for Hispanic Teenage Pregnancy Prevention." *Perspectives on Sexual and Reproductive Health* 36, no. 4 (Summer 2004): 142- 149. https://doi.org/10.1363/3614204.

- Santelli, John, Mary A. Ott, Maureen Lyon, Jennifer Rogers, Daniel Summers, and Rebecca Schleifer. "Abstinence and abstinence-only education: a review of U.S. policies and programs." *Journal of Adolescent Health* 38, no. 1 (January 2006): 72-81. https://doi.org/10.1016/j.jadohealth.2005.10.006.

- *Science and Its Times: Understanding the Social Significance of Scientific Discovery,* s.v. "The Study of Human Sexuality." Accessed August 21, 2020, https://www.encyclopedia.com/science/encyclopedias-almanacs-transcripts-and-maps/study-human-sexuality.

- SIECUS. "A History of AOUM Funding." 2019. https://siecus.org/resources/a-history-of-abstinence-only-federal-funding/.

- SIECUS. "Our History." Accessed August 31, 2020. https://siecus.org/about-siecus/our-history/.

- Trenholm, Christopher, Barbara Devaney, Ken Fortson, Lisa Quay, Justin Wheeler, and Melissa Clark. *Impacts of Four Title V, Section 510 Abstinence Education Programs.* Princeton, NJ: Mathematica Policy Research, 2007. Accessed May 30, 2020. https://www.mathematica.org/our-publications-and-findings/publications/impacts-of-four-title-v-section-510-abstinence-education-programs.

- Underhill, Kristen, Paul Montgomery, and Don Operario. "Sexual abstinence only programmes to prevent HIV infection in high income countries: systematic review." *BMJ* 335, no. 7613 (August 2007): 1-12. https://doi.org/10.1136/bmj.39245.446586.BE.

- Wade, Lisa. *American Hookup: The New Culture of Sex on Campus.* New York: W. W. Norton & Company, 2017.

- Waxman, Henry. "The Content of Federally Funded Abstinence-Only Programs." United States House of Representatives Committee on Government Reform, December 2004. https://spot.colorado.edu/~tooley/HenryWaxman.pdf.

- Weeks, Linton. "When 'Petting Parties' Scandalized The Nation." NPR. May 16, 2015. https://www.npr.org/sections/npr-history-dept/2015/05/26/409126557/when-petting-parties-scandalized-the-nation.

- World Health Organization. *Defining sexual health: Report of a technical consultation on sexual health 28—31 January 2002, Geneva.* Geneva: WHO, 2006. Accessed June 4, 2020. https://www.who.int/reproductivehealth/publications/sexual_health/defining_sexual_health.pdf?ua=1.

Chapter 2

- American Heart Association News. "Why are black women at such high risk of dying from pregnancy complications?" February 20, 2019. https://www.heart.org/en/news/2019/02/20/why-are-black-women-at-such-high-risk-of-dying-from-pregnancy-complications.

- Anson, Pat. "Women in Pain Report Significant Gender Bias." National Pain Report. September 12, 2014. http://nationalpainreport.com/women-in-pain-report-significant-gender-bias-8824696.html.

- *As/Is.* "My Doctor Didn't Believe My Pain." September 2, 2017. Video, 10:05. https://www.youtube.com/watch?v=186OYMYd-3q4&feature=emb_logo.

- Bridges, Khiara M. "Implicit Bias and Racial Disparities in Health Care." American Bar Association. Accessed April 26, 2020. https://www.americanbar.org/groups/crsj/publications/

human_rights_magazine_home/the-state-of-healthcare-in-the-united-states/racial-disparities-in-health-care/.

- Hall, William J., Mimi V. Chapman, Kent M. Lee, Yesenia M. Merino, Tainayah W. Thomas, B. Keith Payne, Eugenia Eng, Steven H. Day, and Tamera Coyne-Beasley. "Implicit Racial/Ethnic Bias Among Health Care Professionals and Its Influence on Health Care Outcomes: A Systematic Review." *American Journal of Public Health* 105, no. 12 (December 2015): 60-76. https://doi.org/10.2105/AJPH.2015.302903.

- Kassebaum, Nicholas J., Ryan M. Barber, Zulfiqar A. Bhutta, Lalit Dandona, Peter W. Gething, Simon I. Hay, Yohannes Kinfu, et al. "Global, regional, and national levels of maternal mortality, 1990—2015: a systematic analysis for the Global Burden of Disease Study 2015," *Lancet* 388, 10053 (October 2016): 1775-1812https://doi.org/10.1016/S0140-6736(16)31470-2

- Mayo Clinic. "Endometriosis." Accessed September 1, 2020. https://www.mayoclinic.org/diseases-conditions/endometriosis/symptoms-causes/syc-20354656.

- McMillan Cottom, Tressie. *Thick: And Other Essays*. New York: The New Press, 2019.

- Pagán, Camille Noe. "When Doctors Downplay Women's Health Concerns." *New York Times*, May 3, 2018. https://www.nytimes.com/2018/05/03/well/live/when-doctors-downplay-womens-health-concerns.html.

- Petersen, Emily E., Nicole L. Davis, David Goodman, Shanna Cox, Carla Syverson, Kristi Seed, Carrie Shapiro-Mendoza, William M. Callaghan, and Wanda Barfield, "Racial/Ethnic Disparities in Pregnancy-Related Deaths — United States, 2007—2016," *Morbidity and Mortality Weekly Report* 68, no. 35 (September 2019): 762-765. http://dx.doi.org/10.15585/mmwr.mm6835a3.

Chapter 4

- Aetna. "Uterine Nerve Ablation (UNA) and Presacral Neurectomy (PSN)." Last modified December 4, 2019. http://www.aetna.com/cpb/medical/data/700_799/0754.html.

- Cleveland Clinic. "Endometriosis: Recurrence and Surgical Management." Last modified August 1, 2014. https://my.clevelandclinic.org/health/diseases/4551-endometriosis-recurrence—surgical-management.

- Endometriosis.net. "How is Endometriosis Treated?" July 5, 2018. https://endometriosis.net/treatment/.

- Guo, Sun-Wei. "Recurrence of endometriosis and its control." *Human Reproduction Update* 15, no. 4 (March 2009): 441-461. https://doi.org/10.1093/humupd/dmp007.

- Health Service Executive. "Vaginismus." Accessed June 15, 2020. https://www.hse.ie/eng/health/az/v/vaginismus/treating-vaginismus.html.

- Kukla, Michelle. "Vaginismus: What It Is and How It Can Be Treated." Good Therapy. March 27, 2018. https://www.

goodtherapy.org/blog/vaginismus-what-it-is-how-it-can-be-treated-0327184.

- Mayo Clinic. "Pap smear." Accessed October 2, 2020. https://www.mayoclinic.org/tests-procedures/pap-smear/about/pac-20394841.

- Moynihan, Erin. "I Have Vaginismus And It Makes Sex So Painful It Feels Like 'Shark Week' In My Vagina." Huffpost. Accessed October 2, 2020. https://www.huffpost.com/entry/vaginismus-painful-sex_n_5bfec73ee4b075d28760a49d.

- National Health Service. "What is cervical screening?" Accessed October 2, 2020. https://www.nhs.uk/conditions/cervical-screening/.

- National Institute of Health, "How do healthcare providers diagnose endometriosis?" Last modified February 21, 2020. https://www.nichd.nih.gov/health/topics/endometri/conditioninfo/diagnose.

- Parker, Lara. "I Stopped Lying About How Happy I Was On Instagram And Started Telling The Truth About Chronic Pain." Buzzfeed. March 7, 2016. https://www.buzzfeed.com/laraparker/i-was-honest-on-instagram-about-my-chronic-pain.

- Parker, Lara. "Learning To Love Life Without Sex." Buzzfeed. April 24, 2014. https://www.buzzfeed.com/laraparker/learning-to-love-life-without-sex.

- Parker, Lara. "What It's Like To Date When You Can't Have Sex." Buzzfeed News. November 15, 2015. https://www.buzzfeednews.com/article/laraparker/what-its-like-to-date-when-you-cant-have-sex.

- Silva, Joana Cavaco. "How to prevent endometriosis pain during sex." Medical News Today. April 6, 2018.https://www.medicalnewstoday.com/articles/321417.

- The American College of Obstetricians and Gynecologists. "Hysterectomy." Accessed June 20, 2020. https://www.acog.org/patient-resources/faqs/special-procedures/hysterectomy.

- University of Michigan. "Laparoscopic Surgery for Endometriosis." Michigan Medicine. Last modified November 7, 2019. https://www.uofmhealth.org/health-library/hw101171.

- University of Pennsylvania. "How the Mayo Clinic Built Its Reputation as a Top Hospital." August 28, 2018. https://knowledge.wharton.upenn.edu/article/mayo-clinics-secret-success/.

- Vaginismus Awareness. Accessed October 2, 2020. http://www.vaginismusawareness.com.

- Vaginismus Network. "Smear Tests." Accessed October 2, 2020. https://www.thevaginismusnetwork.com/smear-tests.

- Vaginismus Network. "The Vaginismus Network's Guide to Smear Tests." Accessed October 2, 2020. https://static1.squarespace.com/static/59c5638df9a61e78f-d5e0713/t/5c5d9532085229cff8237d7c/1549636914700/VN+-Smear+Test+Guide+.pdf.

Chapter 5

- Arnold, Lauren D., Gloria A. Bachmann, Raymond Rosen, and George G. Rhoads. "Assessment of Vulvodynia Symptoms in

a Sample of U.S. Women: A Prevalence Survey with a Nested
Case Control Study." *American Journal of Obstetrics and Gynecology* 196, no. 2 (February 2007): 1-6. https://doi.org/10.1016/j.
ajog.2006.07.047.

- Harlow, Bernard L. and Elizabeth Gunther Stewart. "A
  population-based assessment of chronic unexplained
  vulvar pain: have we underestimated the prevalence of
  vulvodynia?" *Journal of the American Medical Women's Association* 58, no. 2 (January 2003): 82-88. https://
  www.researchgate.net/publication/10762976_A_population-based_assessment_of_chronic_unexplained_vulvar_
  pain_have_we_underestimated_the_prevalence_of_vulvodynia.

- Kraft, Sy. "Vulvodynia: What you need to know." Medical
  News Today. March 13, 2017. https://www.medicalnewstoday.
  com/articles/189076.

- National Vulvodynia Association. "What is Vulvodynia?"
  Accessed June 14, 2020. https://www.nva.org/what-is-vulvodynia/.

- Seehusen, Dean A., Drew C. Baird, and David V. Bode. "Dyspareunia in Women." *American Family Physician* 90, no. 7
  (October 2014): 465-470. https://www.aafp.org/afp/2014/1001/
  afp20141001p465.pdf.

- The American College of Obstetricians and Gynecologists.
  "Vulvodynia." Accessed June 14, 2020. https://www.acog.org/
  en/Patient%20Resources/FAQs/Gynecologic%20Problems/
  Vulvodynia.

Chapter 6

- Harvard Health Publishing. "Treating premenstrual dysphoric disorder." Last modified July 30, 2019. https://www.health. harvard.edu/womens-health/treating-premenstrual-dysphoric-disorder.

- Healthline. "All About the Luteal Phase of the Menstrual Cycle." Accessed September 8, 2020. https://www.healthline. com/health/womens-health/luteal-phase#what-happens.

- International Association for Premenstrual Disorders. "About PMDD." Last modified March 21, 2019. https://iapmd.org/facts-and-figures.

- International Association for Premenstrual Disorders. "Treatment Options." Last modified March 22, 2017. https://iapmd. org/treatment-options.

- International Association for Premenstrual Disorders. "What is PMDD?" Last modified January 14, 2019. https://iapmd.org/about-pmdd.

- Mesen, Tolga B. and Steven L. Young. "Progesterone and the Luteal Phase: A Requisite to Reproduction." *Obstetrics and Gynecology Clinics of North America* 42, no. 1 (March 2015): 135-151. https://doi.org/10.1016/j.ogc.2014.10.003.

- National Institutes of Health. "Sex hormone-sensitive gene complex linked to premenstrual mood disorder." Medical Xpress. January 3, 2017. https://medicalxpress.com/news/2017-01-sex-hormone-sensitive-gene-complex-linked.html.

- Raffi, Edwin R. and Marlene P. Freeman. "The etiology of premenstrual dysphoric disorder: 5 interwoven pieces." *Current Psychiatry* 16, no. 9 (September 2017): 20-28. https://cdn.mdedge.com/files/s3fs-public/Document/August-2017/CP01609020.PDF.

- Schmidt, Peter J., Lynnette K. Nieman, Merry A. Danaceau, Linda F. Adams, and David R. Rubinow. "Differential behavioral effects of gonadal steroids in women with and in those without premenstrual syndrome." *New England Journal of Medicine* 338, no. 4 (January 1998): 209-216. https://doi.org/10.1056/NEJM199801223380401.

Chapter 7

- American Psychiatric Association. *Diagnostic And Statistical Manual Of Mental Disorders, Fifth Edition*. Washington, DC: APA Press, 2013.

- Bertone-Johnson, Elizabeth R., Brian W. Whitcomb, Stacey A. Missmer, JoAnn E. Manson, Susan E. Hankinson, and Janet W. Rich-Edwards. "Early life emotional, physical, and sexual abuse and the development of premenstrual syndrome: a longitudinal study." *Journal of Women's Health* 23, no. 9 (September 2014): 729-739. https://doi.org/10.1089/jwh.2013.4674.

- Holmes, Emily A., Catherine Crane, Melanie J. V. Fennell, and J. Mark G. Williams. "Imagery about suicide in depression—"Flash-forwards"?" *Journal of Behavior Therapy and Experimental Psychiatry* 38, no. 4 (December 2007): 423-434. https://doi.org/10.1016/j.jbtep.2007.10.004.

- Libby, Lisa K., Eric M. Shaeffer, Richard P. Eibach, and Jonathan A. Slemmer. "Picture yourself at the polls: visual perspective in mental imagery affects self-perception and behavior." *Psychological Science* 18, no. 3 (March 2007): 199-203. https://doi.org/10.1111/j.1467-9280.2007.01872.x.

- Mayo Clinic. "Menorrhagia (heavy menstrual bleeding)." Accessed May 15, 2020. https://www.mayoclinic.org/diseases-conditions/menorrhagia/symptoms-causes/syc-20352829.

- McDonald, Fiona. "Scientists Think They Might Have Figured Out The Cause of Severe PMS." Science Alert, January 5, 2017. https://www.sciencealert.com/scientists-think-they-ve-finally-figured-out-the-cause-of-severe-pms-mood-swings.

- Ng, Roger M.K., Martina Di Simplicio, Freda McManus, Helen Kennerley, and Emily A. Holmes. "'Flash-forwards' and suicidal ideation: A prospective investigation of mental imagery, entrapment and defeat in a cohort from the Hong Kong Mental Morbidity Survey." *Psychiatry Research* 246, no. 30 (December 2016): 453-460. https://doi.org/10.1016/j.psychres.2016.10.018.

- Pilver, Corey E., Becca R. Levy, Daniel J. Libby, and Rani A. Desai. "Posttraumatic stress disorder and trauma characteristics are correlates of premenstrual dysphoric disorder." *Archives of Women's Mental Health* 14, no. 5 (July 2011): 383-393. https://doi.org/10.1007/s00737-011-0232-4.

- Raffi, Edwin R. and Marlene P. Freeman. "The etiology of premenstrual dysphoric disorder: 5 interwoven pieces." *Current Psychiatry* 16, no. 9 (September 2017): 20-28. https://cdn.mdedge.com/files/s3fs-public/Document/August-2017/CP01609020.PDF.

Chapter 8

- Grooms, Autumn. "Extra Effort: Tomah's Trista McGovern accepts every challenge, is a role model." *La Crosse Tribune*, March 19, 2011. https://lacrossetribune.com/news/local/education/extra-effort-tomahs-trista-mcgovern-accepts-every-challenge-is-a-role-model/article_8a36673a-4f1c-11e0-8c4d-001cc4c002e0.html.

- McGovern, Trista. "Dismantling What We've Been Told About Disability and Sexuality." The Mighty. December 27, 2019. https://themighty.com/2019/12/trista-mcgovern-disability-sex-positive-photoshoot/.

- McGovern, Trista. Instagram. February 22, 2020. https://www.instagram.com/p/B83zeOcH-5-/.

Chapter 9

- American College of Obstetricians and Gynecologists. "Reproductive Health Care for Women With Disabilities." Powerpoint Presentation. 2010. https://www.aucd.org/docs/ncbddd/webinar/AUCD%20Presentation%20%206-16.pdf.

- Association of State and Territorial Health Officials. *Access to Preventive Healthcare Services for Women with Disabilities*. Arlington, VA: Association of State and Territorial Health Officials, 2013. Accessed June 22, 2020. https://www.astho.org/Access-to-Preventive-Healthcare-Services-for-Women-with-Disabilities-Fact-Sheet/.

- Boni-Saenz, Alexander. "Sexuality and Incapacity." *IIT Chicago-Kent College of Law* 76, no. 6 (September 2015): 1201-1253. https://scholarship.kentlaw.iit.edu/fac_schol/846.

- Centers for Disease Control and Prevention. "Disability Impacts All of Us." Accessed June 22, 2020. https://www.cdc. gov/ncbddd/disabilityandhealth/infographic-disability-impacts-all.html.

- Clarke, Lara. "I've Never Been Catcalled, and I Don't Know How to Feel about it." Medium. April 23, 2020. https://medium. com/conscious-life/ive-never-been-catcalled-and-i-don-t-know-how-to-feel-about-it-af6cecca6cdf.

- Clarke, Tanisha. "Disability Rights and Sexual Health." Association of Maternal & Child Health Programs. Accessed June 16, 2020. http://www.amchp.org/AboutAMCHP/Newsletters/Pulse/NovDec17/Pages/Disability-Rights-and-Sexual-Health. aspx.

- Horner-Johnson, Willi, Konrad Dobbertin, Elena M. Andresen, and Lisa I Iezzoni. "Breast and cervical cancer screening disparities associated with disability severity." *Women's Health Issues* 24, no. 1 (January 2014): 147-153. https://doi.org/10.1016/j. whi.2013.10.009.

- Iezzoni, Lisa I., Stephen G. Kurtz, and Sowmya R. Rao. "Trends in Mammography Over Time for Women With and Without Chronic Disability." *Journal of Women's Health* 24, no. 7 (July 2015): 593-601. https://doi.org/10.1089/jwh.2014.5181.

- Iezzoni, Lisa I., Stephen G. Kurtz, and Sowmya R. Rao. "Trends in Pap Testing Over Time for Women With and Without Chronic Disability," *American Journal of Preventative Medicine* 50, no. 2 (February 2016): 210-219. https://doi.org/10.1016/j. amepre.2015.06.031.

- Mahmoudi, Elham and Michelle A. Meade. "Disparities in access to health care among adults with physical disabilities: analysis of a representative national sample for a ten-year period." *Disability and Health Journal* 8, no. 2 (April 2015): 182-190. https://doi.org/10.1016/j.dhjo.2014.08.007.

- McColl, Mary Ann, Donna Forster, S. E. D. Shortt, Duncan Hunter, John Dorland, Marshall Godwin, and Walter Rosser. "Physician Experiences Providing Primary Care to People with Disabilities." *Healthcare Policy* 4, no. 1 (August 2008): 129-147. https://www.ncbi.nlm.nih.gov/pmc/articles/PMC2645198/pdf/policy-04-e129.pdf.

- Silvers, Anita, Leslie Francis, and Brittany Badesch. "Reproductive Rights and Access to Reproductive Services for Women with Disabilities." *American Medical Association Journal of Ethics* 18, no. 4 (April 2016): 430-437. https://journalofethics.ama-assn.org/article/reproductive-rights-and-access-reproductive-services-women-disabilities/2016-04.

- Wright, Elizabeth. "Devoted to Disability: are devotees really that creepy?" Medium. May 6, 2020. https://medium.com/conscious-life/devoted-to-disability-are-devotees-really-that-creepy-75514ead4914.

- Wright, Elizabeth. "Infantilising Disabled People is a Thing and You're Probably Unconsciously Doing It." Medium. January 13, 2020. https://medium.com/age-of-awareness/infantilising-disabled-people-is-a-thing-and-youre-probably-unconsciously-doing-it-1adf91dc0fc5.

- Yates, Emily. "'Pretty Cripples' and the people turned on by disability." BBC. March 12, 2016. https://www.bbc.com/news/disability-35762887.

Chapter 10

- American Civil Liberties Union. "Schroer v. Billington." Accessed September 7, 2020. https://www.acludc.org/en/cases/schroer-v-billington.

- Bauer, Greta R., Rebecca Hammond, Robb Travers, Matthias Kaay, Karin M Hohenadel, and Michelle Boyce. ""I don't think this is theoretical; this is our lives": how erasure impacts health care for transgender people." *Journal of the Association of Nurses in AIDS Care* 20, no. 5 (September-October 2009): 348-361. https://doi.org/10.1016/j.jana.2009.07.004.

- Blair, Karen L. and Rhea A. Hoskin. "Transgender exclusion from the world of dating: Patterns of acceptance and rejection of hypothetical trans dating partners as a function of sexual and gender identity." *Journal of Social and Personal Relationships* 34, no. 7 (May 2018): 2074-2095. https://doi.org/10.1177/0265407518779139.

- Cornell Law School. "But-for test." Legal Information Institute. Accessed September 7, 2020. https://www.law.cornell.edu/wex/but-for_test.

- Ennis, Dawn. "10 Words Transgender People Want You to Know (But Not Say)." Advocate. February 4, 2016. https://www.advocate.com/transgender/2016/1/19/10-words-transgender-people-want-you-know-not-say.

- Gender Minorities. "Trans 101: Glossary of Trans Words and How to Use Them." Accessed October 3, 2020. https://gender-minorities.com/database/glossary-transgender/.

- Grant, Jaime M., Lisa A. Mottet, Justin Tanis, Jack Harrison, Jody L. Herman, and Mara Keisling. *Injustice at Every Turn: A Report of the National Transgender Discrimination Survey.* Washington DC: National Center for Transgender Equality and National Gay and Lesbian Task Force, 2011. Accessed June 8, 2020. https://www.transequality.org/sites/default/files/docs/resources/NTDS_Report.pdf.

- Holden, Alexandra. "The Gay/Trans Panic Defense: What It is, and How to End It." American Bar Association. April 1, 2020. https://www.americanbar.org/groups/crsj/publications/member-features/gay-trans-panic-defense/.

- Human Rights Campaign. "Understanding the Transgender Community." Accessed October 6, 2020. https://www.hrc.org/resources/understanding-the-transgender-community.

- James, Sandy E., Jody L. Herman, Susan Rankin, Mara Keisling, Lisa Mottet, and Ma'ayan Anafi. *The Report of the 2015 U.S. Transgender Survey.* Washington, DC: National Center for Transgender Equality, 2016. Accessed June 8, 2020. https://www.transequality.org/sites/default/files/docs/usts/USTS%20Full%20Report%20-%20FINAL%201.6.17.pdf.

- Juzwiak, Rich. "Am I Fetishizing Trans Women as a Cis Guy Who Seeks Them Out for Sex?" Slate. August 21, 2019. https://slate.com/human-interest/2019/08/trans-chasing-for-cis-guy-to-seek-women-for-sex.html.

- Keuroghlian, Alex S., Kevin L. Ard, and Harvey J. Makadon. "Advancing health equity for lesbian, gay, bisexual and transgender (LGBT) people through sexual health education and LGBT-affirming health care environments." *Sexual Health* 14, (February 2017): 119-122. http://dx.doi.org/10.1071/SH16145.

- Lang, Nico. "Looking for Love and Acceptance: Dating While Trans in America." Daily Beast. Last modified July 12, 2017. https://www.thedailybeast.com/looking-for-love-and-acceptance-dating-while-trans-in-america.

- Madison, Mila. "Transgender Fetishism and the Culture of Chasers." Maven. September 19, 2016. https://mavenroundtable.io/transgenderuniverse/articles/transgender-fetishism-and-the-culture-of-chasers-YoMo3y-7WhEqocwIZhhmrXA.

- Mamone, Tris. "For Trans Men Seeking Reproductive Health Care, 'There Are Barriers Every Step of the Way'." *Rewire.News*, July 3, 2019. https://rewire.news/article/2019/07/03/trans-men-reproductive-health-care/.

- Milloy, Christin S. "Beware the Chasers: "Admirers" Who Harass Trans People." Slate. October 2, 2014. https://slate.com/human-interest/2014/10/trans-chasers-exploitive-admirers-who-harass-trans-people.html.

- Penn State Student Affairs. "Gender Diversity Terminology." Accessed October 3, 2020. https://studentaffairs.psu.edu/campus-community-diversity/lgbtq-community/explore-lgbtq-resources/identity-based-resources/gender-terms.

- Reign, Eva. "Trans Women and Femmes Speak Out About Being Fetishized." Them. July 21, 2018. https://www.them.us/story/trans-women-femmes-fetishization.

- Serano, Julia. *Whipping Girl: A Transsexual Woman on Sexism and the Scapegoating of Femininity.* Seal Press, 2016.

- *Story District.* "Morgan Givens in Story District's Emotional Overload on August 11, 2015." September 8, 2015. Video, 9:58. https://www.youtube.com/watch?time_continue=346&v=pVs1e_JCuaU&feature=emb_title.

- *Story District.* "Morgan Givens in Story District's Top Shelf." February 4, 2016. Video, 10:16. https://www.youtube.com/watch?time_continue=250&v=N8z2gU7v6R0&feature=emb_title.

- Tannehill, Brynn. "Is Refusing to Date Trans People Transphobic?" Advocate. December 14, 2019. https://www.advocate.com/commentary/2019/12/14/refusing-date-trans-people-transphobic.

Chapter 11

- AHA Foundation. "Vacation Cutting: An Illegal Practice Still Running Rampant." Accessed June 18, 2020. https://www.theahafoundation.org/vacation-cutting-an-illegal-practice-still-running-rampant/.

- Amnesty International. "What is Female Genital Mutilation?" Accessed March 27, 2020. https://www.amnesty.org/download/Documents/156000/act770051997en.pdf.

- Baker, Aryn. "Doctors Around the World Rally for New Surgery to Counter Female Genital Mutilation." *Time*, March 21, 2017. https://time.com/4707899/victims-of-fgm-see-new-hope-in-life-changing-surgery/.

- Bergstrom, Renee. "FGM happened to me in white, midwest America." The Guardian. December 3, 2016. https://www.theguardian.com/us-news/2016/dec/02/fgm-happened-to-me-in-white-midwest-america.

- Fortin, Jacey. "Michigan Doctor Is Accused of Genital Cutting of 2 Girls." *The New York Times*, April 13, 2017. https://www.nytimes.com/2017/04/13/us/michigan-doctor-fgm-cutting.html?_r=0.

- Goldberg, Howard, Paul Stupp, Ekwutosi Okoroh, Ghenet Besera, David Goodman, and Isabella Danel. "Female Genital Mutilation/Cutting in the United States: Updated Estimates of Women and Girls at Risk, 2012." *Public Health Reports* 131, no. 2 (March-April 2016): 340-347. https://doi.org/10.1177/003335491613100218.

- History. "U.S. Immigration Since 1965." Last modified June 7, 2019. https://www.history.com/topics/immigration/us-immigration-since-1965.

- Kamali-Nafar, Soraya. "Why FGM in the US is Rarely Prosecuted." Women In International Security. July 13, 2018. https://www.wiisglobal.org/why-fgm-in-the-us-is-rarely-prosecuted/.

- Karimjee, Mariya. "Who Do We Think We Are?" *This American Life.* May 6, 2016. https://www.thisamericanlife.org/586/who-do-we-think-we-are.

- Lalla-Maharajh, Julia. "Female Genital Mutilation in Georgia, USA." HuffPost. Last modified December 6, 2017. https://www.huffpost.com/entry/female-genital-mutilation_b_498529?guccounter=1.

- Lobo, Maria. "Consider the potential emotional and psychological consequences of female genital mutilation." Senior Thesis, Imperial College London. Accessed October 6, 2020. https://www.rcpsych.ac.uk/docs/default-source/members/faculties/perinatal-psychiatry/perinatal-prizes-lobo.pdf?sfvrsn=c-2d14c5d_2.

- Mather, Mark and Charlotte Feldman-Jacobs. "Women and Girls at Risk of Female Genital Mutilation/Cutting in the United States." PRB. February 5, 2016. https://www.prb.org/us-fgmc/.

- McCallum, Annie. "LaGrange crime: Woman charged with female genital mutilation, 2nd-degree cruelty to children." *Ledger-Enquirer.* Last modified March 11, 2010. https://www.ledger-enquirer.com/news/local/article29124460.html.

- Miller, Michael and Francesca Moneti. *Changing a Harmful Social Convention: Female Genital Mutilation/Cutting.* Florence, Italy: UNICEF, 2008. Accessed March 27, 2020. https://www.unicef-irc.org/publications/pdf/fgm_eng.pdf.

- Moghe, Sonia. "3 US women share the horrors of female genital mutilation." CNN. May 11, 2017. https://www.cnn.com/2017/05/11/health/fgm-us-survivor-stories-trnd/index.html.

- Pyati, Archana and Claudia De Palma. *Female Genital Mutilation: Protecting Girls and Women in the U.S. from FGM and Vacation Cutting.* New York: Sanctuary for Families, 2013. Accessed March 27, 2020. https://www.sanctuaryforfamilies.org/wp-content/uploads/sites/18/2015/07/FGM-Report-March-2013.pdf.

- Raja, Tasneem. "I Underwent Genital Mutilation as a Child—Right Here in the United States." *Mother Jones*, April 21, 2017. https://www.motherjones.com/politics/2017/04/genital-cutting-indian-doctor-women-khatna/.

- Tasneem Raja. Interview by Ari Shapiro and Audie Cornish. *All Things Considered.* NPR. April 24, 2017. https://www.npr.org/2017/04/24/525441611/writer-recalls-undergoing-female-genital-mutilation-in-the-u-s.

- Taher, Mariya. "The Duality of My Life: Growing Up a Hybrid of American and Dawoodi Bohra." *Brown Girl Magazine*, January 10, 2018. https://www.browngirlmagazine.com/2018/01/the-duality-of-my-life/.

- The Dawoodi Bohras. "Attire & Tradition." Accessed March 27, 2020. https://www.thedawoodibohras.com/culture/attire-tradition/.

- The Dawoodi Bohras. "The Bohras Today." Accessed March 27, 2020. https://www.thedawoodibohras.com/about-the-bohras/the-bohras-today/.

- The Dawoodi Bohras. "The Da'I Al-Mutlaq." Accessed March 27, 2020. https://www.thedawoodibohras.com/about-the-bohras/the-dai-al-mutlaq/.

- Tucker, Matthew. "These British Women Are All Survivors Of Female Genital Mutilation." Buzzfeed News. July 16, 2016. https://www.buzzfeed.com/matthewtucker/these-british-women-are-all-survivors-of-female-genital-muti.

- United Nations Population Fund. "Female genital mutilation." Accessed March 27, 2020. https://www.unfpa.org/female-genital-mutilation.

- Wescott, Lucy. "Female Genital Mutilation on the Rise in the U.S." Newsweek. February 6, 2015. https://www.newsweek.com/fgm-rates-have-doubled-us-2004-304773.

- World Health Organization. "Female genital mutilation." Last modified February 3, 2020. https://www.who.int/news-room/fact-sheets/detail/female-genital-mutilation.

- Zoeb, Mariya. "Happy Threads — Know Our World." The Dawoodi Bohras. November 8, 2019. https://www.thedawoodibohras.com/2019/11/08/happy-threads-know-our-world/.

Chapter 12

- Baldwin, Aleta, Brian Dodge, Vanessa R. Schick, Brenda Light, Phillip W. Schnarrs, Debby Herbenick, and J. Dennis Fortenberry. "Transgender and Genderqueer Individuals' Experiences with Health Care Providers: What's Working, What's Not, and Where Do We Go from Here?" *Journal of Health Care for the Poor and Underserved* 29, no. 4 (November 2018): 1300-1318. doi: 10.1353/hpu.2018.0097.

- Boskey, Elizabeth. "What Does It Mean to Be Non-Binary or Have Non-Binary Gender?" Very Well Mind. September 28, 2019. https://www.verywellmind.com/what-does-it-mean-to-be-non-binary-or-have-non-binary-gender-4172702#citation-5.

- *Dictionary.com.* S.v. "male gaze." Accessed September 9, 2020. https://www.dictionary.com/browse/male-gaze.

- Harris-Perry, Melissa V. *Sister Citizen: Shame, Stereotypes, and Black Women in America.* New Haven: Yale University Press, 2011.

- Human Rights Campaign. "Bisexual Health Awareness Month: Mental Health in the Bisexual Community." March 24, 2017. https://www.hrc.org/news/bisexual-health-awareness-month-mental-health-in-the-bisexual-community.

- Jacobsson, Eva-Maria. *A Female Gaze?* Stockholm, Sweden: KTH Royal Institute of Technology, 1999. Accessed September 9, 2020. http://citeseerx.ist.psu.edu/viewdoc/download;jsessionid=461FED3025C945411C9BAAB-99364C5E9?doi=10.1.1.29.2891&rep=rep1&type=pdf.

- James, Sandy E., Jody L. Herman, Susan Rankin, Mara Keisling, Lisa Mottet, and Ma'ayan Anafi. *The Report of the 2015 U.S. Transgender Survey.* Washington, DC: National Center for Transgender Equality, 2016. Accessed June 8, 2020. https://www.transequality.org/sites/default/files/docs/usts/USTS%20Full%20Report%20-%20FINAL%201.6.17.pdf.

- Jimenez, Jorge A. and José M. Abreu. "Race and sex effects on attitudinal perceptions of acquaintance rape." *Journal of Counseling Psychology* 50, no. 2 (2003): 252-256. https://doi.org/10.1037/0022-0167.50.2.252.

- Jost, John T., Mahzarin R. Banaji, and Brian A. Nosek. "A Decade of System Justification Theory: Accumulated Evidence of Conscious and Unconscious Bolstering of the Status Quo." *Political Psychology* 25, no. 6 (December 2004): 881-919. https://doi.org/10.1111/j.1467-9221.2004.00402.x.

- Joyal, Christian C., Amelie Cossette, and Vanessa LaPierre. "What is an unusual sexual fantasy?" *Journal of Sexual Medicine* 12 (2015): 328-340.

- Kiesel, Laura. "My First Lap — Part 1," Endometriosis.net, July 23, 2018. https://endometriosis.net/living/first-lap-part-1/.

- Kiesel, Laura. "The Burden of Invisible Illness." Medium. December 16, 2018. https://medium.com/s/for-the-record/the-burden-of-invisible-illness-just-because-i-dont-look-disabled-doesn-t-mean-i-m-not-7d0be07bb09b.

- Lamb, Sharon, Tangela Roberts, and Aleksandra Plocha. *Girls of Color, Sexuality, and Sex Education.* New York: Palgrave Macmillan, 2016.

- Losty, Mairéad and John O'Connor. "Falling outside of the 'nice little binary box': a psychoanalytic exploration of the non-binary gender identity." *Psychoanalytic Psychotherapy* 32, no. 1 (October 2017): 40-60. https://doi.org/10.1080/02668734 .2017.1384933.

- Lykens, James E., Allen J. LeBlanc, and Walter O. Bockting. "Healthcare Experiences Among Young Adults Who Identify as Genderqueer or Nonbinary." *LGBT Health* 5, no. 3 (April 2018): 191-196. https://doi.org/10.1089/lgbt.2017.0215.

- Magill, Elizabeth. "Medical Schools Failing at Pain Education." National Pain Report. April 16, 2012. http://nationalpainreport. com/medical-schools-failing-at-pain-education-8813868.html.

- McDowell, Michal J. and Iman K. Berrahou. *Learning to Address Implicit Bias Toward LGBTQ Patients: Case Scenarios.* Boston, MA: National LGBT Health Education Center, 2018. Accessed April 26, 2020. https://www.lgbtqiaheal-theducation.org/wp-content/uploads/2018/10/Implicit-Bias-Guide-2018_Final.pdf.

- Rupp, Kalman. "Factors Affecting Initial Disability Allowance Rates for the Disability Insurance and Supplemental Security Income Programs: The Role of the Demographic and Diagnostic Composition of Applicants and Local Labor Market Conditions." *Social Security Bulletin* 72, no. 4 (November 2012): 11-35. https://ssrn.com/abstract=2172488.

- Sabin, Janice A., Rachel G. Riskind, and Brian A. Nosek. "Health Care Providers' Implicit and Explicit Attitudes Toward Lesbian Women and Gay Men." *American Journal of Public Health* 105, no. 9 (September 2015): 1831-1841. https://doi.org/10.2105/AJPH.2015.302631.

- Scandurra, Cristiano, Fabrizio Mezza, Nelson Mauro Maldonato, Mario Bottone, Vincenzo Bochicchio, Paolo Valerio, and Roberto Vitelli. "Health of Non-binary and Genderqueer People: A Systematic Review." *Frontiers in Psychology* 10, no. 1453 (June 2019): 1-12. https://doi.org/10.3389/fpsyg.2019.01453.

- Scanlon, Julie and Ruth Lewis. "Whose Sexuality Is It Anyway? Women's Experiences of Viewing Lesbians on Screen." *Feminist Media Studies* 17, no. 6 (2017): 1005-1021. http://dx.doi.org/10.1080/14680777.2016.1257998.

- Villarosa, Linda. "Myths about physical racial differences were used to justify slavery — and are still believed by doctors today." *The New York Times Magazine*, August 14, 2019. https://www.nytimes.com/interactive/2019/08/14/magazine/racial-differences-doctors.html.

- Wong, May. "Q&A: What's behind the gender gap in disability benefits?" Stanford Institute for Economic Policy Research (SIEPR). April 1, 2020. https://siepr.stanford.edu/news/gender-gap-disability-benefits.

Chapter 13

- Allahdadi, Kyan J., Rita C.A. Tostes, and R. Clinton Webb. "Female Sexual Dysfunction: Therapeutic Options and Experimental Challenges." *Cardiovasc Hematol Agents Med Chem* 7, no. 4 (October 2009): 260-269. https://www.eurekaselect.com/70234/article.

- Clancy, Carolyn M. and Charlea T. Massion. "American Women's Health Care: A Patchwork Quilt With Gaps." *JAMA* 268, no. 14 (1992). Quoted in Pamela Karney. "Women's Health: An Evolving Mosaic." *Journal of General Internal Medicine* 15, no. 8 (August 2000): 600-602. https://doi.org/10.1046/j.1525-1497.2000.00623.x.

- Mayo Clinic. "Female Sexual Dysfunction." Accessed September 12, 2020. https://www.mayoclinic.org/diseases-conditions/female-sexual-dysfunction/symptoms-causes/syc-20372549.

- Nichols, Francine H. "History of the Women's Health Movement in the 20th Century." *Journal of Obstetric, Gynecologic, & Neonatal Nursing* 29, no. 1 (June 1999): 56-64. https://doi.org/10.1111/j.1552-6909.2000.tb02756.x.